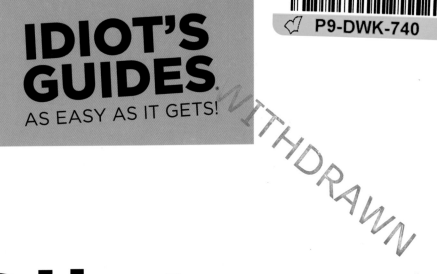

IDIOT'S GUIDES
AS EASY AS IT GETS!

Pilates

by Linda Paden, DPT

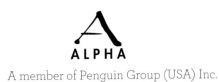

ALPHA

A member of Penguin Group (USA) Inc.

ALPHA BOOKS

Published by Penguin Group (USA) Inc.

Penguin Group (USA) Inc., 375 Hudson Street, New York, New York 10014, USA • Penguin Group (Canada), 90 Eglinton Avenue East, Suite 700, Toronto, Ontario M4P 2Y3, Canada (a division of Pearson Penguin Canada Inc.) • Penguin Books Ltd., 80 Strand, London WC2R 0RL, England • Penguin Ireland, 25 St. Stephen's Green, Dublin 2, Ireland (a division of Penguin Books Ltd.) • Penguin Group (Australia), 250 Camberwell Road, Camberwell, Victoria 3124, Australia (a division of Pearson Australia Group Pty. Ltd.) • Penguin Books India Pvt. Ltd., 11 Community Centre, Panchsheel Park, New Delhi—110 017, India • Penguin Group (NZ), 67 Apollo Drive, Rosedale, North Shore, Auckland 1311, New Zealand (a division of Pearson New Zealand Ltd.) • Penguin Books (South Africa) (Pty.) Ltd., 24 Sturdee Avenue, Rosebank, Johannesburg 2196, South Africa • Penguin Books Ltd., Registered Offices: 80 Strand, London WC2R 0RL, England

IDIOT'S GUIDES and Design are trademarks of Penguin Group (USA) Inc.

International Standard Book Number: 978-1-61564-651-7
Library of Congress Catalog Card Number: 2014941121

16 15 14   8 7 6 5 4 3 2 1

Interpretation of the printing code: The rightmost number of the first series of numbers is the year of the book's printing; the rightmost number of the second series of numbers is the number of the book's printing. For example, a printing code of 14-1 shows that the first printing occurred in 2014.

Note: This publication contains the opinions and ideas of its author. It is intended to provide helpful and informative material on the subject matter covered. It is sold with the understanding that the author and publisher are not engaged in rendering professional services in the book. If the reader requires personal assistance or advice, a competent professional should be consulted. The author and publisher specifically disclaim any responsibility for any liability, loss, or risk, personal or otherwise, which is incurred as a consequence, directly or indirectly, of the use and application of any of the contents of this book.

Publisher: *Mike Sanders*

Executive Managing Editor: *Billy Fields*

Senior Acquisitions Editor: *Brook Farling*

Development Editor: *Kayla Dugger*

Senior Production Editor: *Janette Lynn*

Cover and Book Designer: *Rebecca Batchelor*

Indexer: *Johnna VanHoose Dinse*

Layout: *Ayanna Lacey*

Proofreader: *Monica Stone*

Contents

Introduction

Whatever your reasons are for reading this book—for your overall fitness, to improve your flexibility, to develop core strength, to develop long and lean muscles, to prevent injury—the exercises described in this book will help you develop healthy movement patterns and a balance of strength and flexibility. The best way to learn Pilates is with a well-trained instructor who can check your technique and form while doing the exercises. That said, I personally started learning Pilates work from a book at home.

Let me share why Pilates is a love of mine. I am your typical Pilates story—a young dancer who got hurt and found Pilates. My mother gave me my first mat Pilates book. At first, I set the book to the side, skeptical that these odd movements would do me any good. But with my mother's patient and consistent suggestion, I started doing a beginner mat program. After doing some basic Pilates mat exercises at home, I started feeling better! I then discovered the spring-resistance Pilates machines in 2003 when a Pilates studio opened in Fort Wayne, Indiana. As I developed a balance of core stability, strength, and flexibility, I felt even better! Once you know what it is like to feel good, there is no going back. In 2003, I started my teacher training and have loved Pilates work ever since.

After watching those who have done Pilates throughout their lives move well into their seventies, eighties, and nineties, it is a testimony to the work. Even with the years I have studied this work, there is still more that I have yet to learn and movement goals I have to reach. With the Pilates work, there is always room to grow.

Also, if you're like many people, you spend so much time focusing on what is going on around you rather than on yourself. Pilates is the time to develop that mind-body connection and focus on how your body is feeling and moving. Enjoy the time to focus on your body and rejuvenate!

As you embark on your adventure of learning Pilates mat work, may you move well.

How to Use This Book

This book has four main parts:

In **Part 1, Pilates Essentials,** you are introduced to the Pilates principles, alignments, and simple movements. This part gives you some basic info to get started and get moving right away.

Part 2, Pilates Mat Exercises, contains a list of mat exercises arranged by body position: on your back, on your side, seated, on your stomach, planks and all fours, and standing.

Part 3, Pilates Equipment Exercises, includes exercises arranged by small equipment you can easily find at a store or even around the house: ring, arm weights, band or pole, large ball, and foam roller.

Finally, **Part 4, Pilates Routines,** contains programs for a good workout. You can do total-body programs, programs that target a certain area of the body, or even programs based on different sports!

I recommend you begin by gaining a good understanding of the material in Chapters 1 to 3. You can then go through the preparatory or beginner programs found in Chapter 15 for direction on which exercises to begin with.

As you are learning the exercises, remember to take your time and only do the exercises that you can do safely. I believe Pilates and the Pilates principles are for everyone, but not every exercise is. If you have a history of injury, consult with your health-care provider before attempting any of the exercises in this book.

Acknowledgments

There are many to thank for the support, help, and knowledge that is found in the book. To the instructors who taught me Pilates work, as well as gave me the knowledge from my academic education, thank you for sharing your wisdom and having a teacher's heart. To Teresa Hunt, for not only opening your studio, Re-Form Movement Pilates, for the photo shoot, but also being a model and technical editor for this project. I love teaching at Re-Form Movement Pilates! Thank you to the other models found throughout this book—Megan Hazelrigg, Carmenza Snider, Molly Palmatier Tittle, and Jerry Denys. To the photographer, Greg Perez, who took the collection of photos for this book. Finally, to those at Alpha Books, including Brook Farling, acquisitions editor; and Kayla Dugger, development editor; and the others involved with this project. Thank you for helping make this book what it is!

To my clients who share their time, attention, and lives since I started teaching Pilates in 2004, thank you for your dedication to Pilates work! I feel blessed to have the opportunity to teach such a lovely group of people. I hope this book may be a resource to help you move and live well.

To my mother, Bernice Gilman, thank you for introducing me to the work and watching me develop my passion.

PART 1

Pilates Essentials

The material in this part sets the foundation for the exercises and programs in the rest of the book. First, you are introduced to Pilates' philosophy and principles. You then learn about alignment to help you start to develop body awareness. I also provide activities to try to get you moving, feeling, and experiencing the benefits of Pilates as quickly as possible. After you understand alignment, I then teach you how to breathe, the Pilates scoop, and basic movements. Once you finish learning these, you'll be ready to explore the rest of the book!

CHAPTER 1

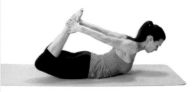

What Is Pilates?

Joseph Pilates called his work *Contrology* and claimed it was "designed to give you suppleness, natural grace, and skill that will be unmistakably reflected in the way you walk, in the way you play, and the way you work." In my experience, his claim has proven true.

This chapter briefly reviews how Pilates work came to be what it is today and introduces the Pilates principles. The Pilates principles should be applied to every Pilates movement and exercise. If you enjoy lists, at the end of this chapter is a short checklist to help you assess how well you are applying the principles to an exercise. The end goal is that every exercise and movement you do will include all six of the principles.

who was joseph pilates?

The founder of the Pilates method, Joseph Pilates, was born in Germany in 1883. What we today call *Pilates*, Joe called *Contrology*. He developed his system of movements after studying movements of animals and Eastern and Western exercise regimens. He used his movements in an intern camp in England during World War I, where he worked with injured soldiers.

In 1926, Joe came to America, where he opened a studio in New York with his wife Clara, whom he had met on the ship over. In New York, he taught his exercises to injured dancers, several of whom went on to teach his work and became known as the elders. For his studio work with his students, Joe designed his own exercise equipment. Many of his apparatuses are being manufactured today, including the cadillac, reformer, chair, ring, ladder barrel, spine corrector, foot corrector, and toe corrector.

Joe wrote two books, *Your Health* in 1934 and *Pilates' Return to Life Through Contrology* in 1945. His later book includes pictures of him doing 34 of his Pilates mat exercises, many of which are also included here in this book. Joe argued that inactive lifestyles did not suffice in maintaining the body or health. He felt his method of exercise would safely challenge the body and wanted to change the world through physical fitness. Passing in 1967, Joe was a man ahead of his time.

WHAT IS THE DIFFERENCE BETWEEN PILATES MAT WORK AND PILATES EQUIPMENT WORK?

Many of the body positions and exercises in this book have variations done using Joe's equipment. Some of the equipment, like the spine corrector and the ladder barrel, are shaped in an arc to help support and stretch the body and spine. Other pieces of equipment—including the cadillac, reformer, and chair—use springs of various tension to provide resistance. Sometimes the springs provide assistance for the exercise, allowing for good technique, deeper core work, or supported stretch. For other exercises, the springs provide resistance for development of strength, power, and endurance. At the time of writing this book, I personally have a reformer, chair, and spine corrector in my living room, in addition to the equipment found throughout this book. Because the machine are so versatile, it is like having an entire gym at home!

philosophy of pilates work

Pilates is more than just a form of exercise; it is a philosophy toward movement. Today, there are a number of "flavors" of Pilates, from traditional to contemporary. However, all of the work comes back to Joseph Pilates' philosophy. I like to explain the variations as flavors of ice cream—although there are many flavors, the ice cream is made up of the same foundational ingredients.

Pilates movements develop a balance of muscle strength, endurance, and flexibility. It does not develop bulky muscles; instead, it develops the long, lean muscles needed for movement in your daily life. These long, lean muscles are also less prone to injury. In addition to developing well-functioning muscles, it teaches you coordination of movement. Pilates exercises focus the work on the core and deep muscles of your body. Once these deep muscles are strong, the superficial, showy muscles will naturally develop.

As each exercise has a breathing pattern, Pilates exercises gently activate the cardiovascular and respiratory systems of your body. The various body positions also encourage the air and blood going to your lungs to enter different sections of your lungs. The benefits can include improved endurance, increased lung capacity, and mental clarity. When the exercises are done correctly, you can feel calm and focused after doing Pilates work.

HOW OFTEN SHOULD YOU DO THE PILATES EXERCISES? HOW QUICKLY CAN YOU EXPECT RESULTS?

These are two of the most common questions I am asked by those new to the Pilates work. Pilates was designed to slowly change your body, posture, and the way you move. In his book, Joseph Pilates suggested four times a week for three months for a transformation of body, mind, and spirit. I agree with his recommendation that doing the Pilates exercises four times a week is most beneficial. However, even if you are unable to do the exercises this frequently, focus on doing what you can correctly. These movements will be beneficial for your body and mind, even if it takes longer to see results.

pilates principles

There are several principles that should be incorporated into every Pilates exercise: centering, concentration, control, precision, breath, and flow of movement.

Centering

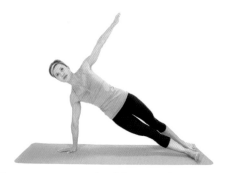

Every movement should initiate from your torso and your core muscles. When your center is stable, your limbs have a foundation on which to move.

Concentration

As Joseph Pilates said, "Not mind *or* body but mind *and* body!" When you do Pilates, take the time to pay attention to the details of your body. Being present mentally when doing Pilates exercises will help you develop a mind-body connection and body awareness.

Control

Every movement should be done with control. Moving with control helps ensure your safety during the exercises by protecting you from injury. Keep in mind, using control does not always mean you move slowly; however, it does mean you always move with purposeful intention.

Precision

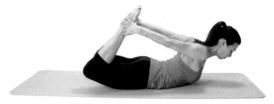

You will find that each exercise has a specific alignment, form, and focus. These directions should be carried out precisely, with attention to the positioning and movements of your entire body. Such attention to detail helps you correct your posture and develop better balance.

Breath

Your core and endurance muscles perform best when they have oxygen. Every Pilates exercise has a matching, continuous breathing pattern with inhalations through your nose and exhalations out your mouth. This gentle respiratory and cardiovascular work in Pilates energizes your body and mind.

Flow of Movement

Flow of movement is your last principle of focus, as it normally requires familiarity with the exercises. Once a group of exercises is learned, you can work on moving from one exercise to another without resting in between. As you go through each exercise in a program, allow yourself to move with poise and grace.

pilates exercises

Before attempting a Pilates exercise, spend some time in the rest of the chapters in this part to learn the proper alignment and positioning of your body and the modified Pilates movements to get you started. The basic movements can be used as exercises until you are ready to begin the mat movements. For now, though, I'd like to give you a general overview of the best way to approach Pilates exercises.

You want to start slowly by performing fewer repetitions and a smaller range of movements. You should stay only within a range of movement where you can maintain good alignment and form. It is okay to stay with an easier version of an exercise. Eventually, you will be able to do larger and more challenging movements. Remember, the philosophy behind Pilates and the exercises is developing healthy movement patterns in the body. Forming new movement habits will take time.

If you ever have pain, repetitive snapping, or something that doesn't feel right during an exercise, stop the movements you are doing. Ignore the cliché, "No pain, no gain." Muscle burn is okay, but you want to avoid pain. When you do Pilates exercises, it is a time to be attentive and listen to your body.

The following are some questions to ask yourself about your approach in relation to each Pilates principle:

- **Centering:** Did the movement initiate from your core?

- **Concentration:** Were you focused on the movement you were doing?

- **Control:** Did you stay within a range where you could use good form?

- **Precision:** Did you pay attention to the details of the movement and alignment?

- **Breath:** Did each movement you perform have a matching breathing pattern?

- **Flow of Movement:** Did you perform the exercise with continuous motion?

As you learn some of the exercises, consider coming back to this list to see how you applied the principles to the exercise.

CHAPTER 2

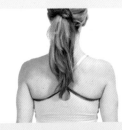

Alignment

In this chapter, you learn how to place the bones of your body, from feet to head, in good alignment. This ties in to the Pilates principle of centering, which is especially important during Pilates mat exercises. Having your center or core well aligned and stable allows for free movement of your arms and legs.

The muscles of your body can't work at their best when placed in a position that is too long or too short. This alignment helps you avoid unnecessary strain on your body and also allows your muscles to be the optimal length.

foot triangles

Find Alignment

Your feet are the base of support for your body when in a standing position. To distribute your body weight evenly, imagine foot triangles on the bottom of your feet. The first point of the triangle is located at the base of your first toe, the second point at the base of your fifth toe, and the last point in the center of the heel. The goal is to have equal pressure in all three points of the triangle when your feet are flat on the floor for Pilates exercises.

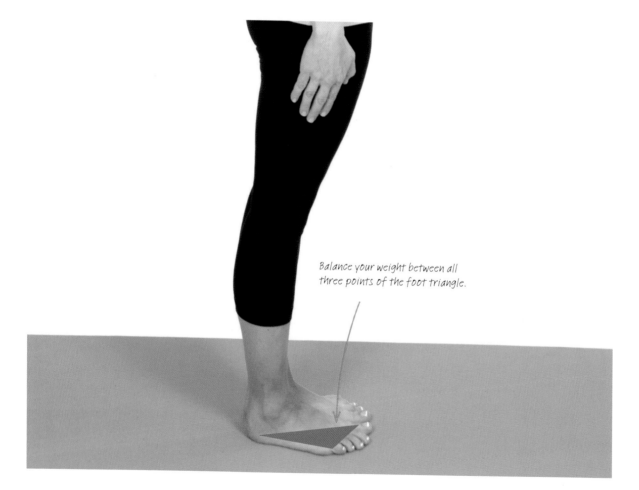

Balance your weight between all three points of the foot triangle.

Practice Activities

Small changes in the weight distribution on the bottom of your feet can impact the alignment of the rest of your body. Try the following activities to understand the difference.

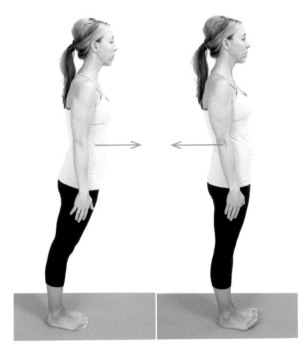

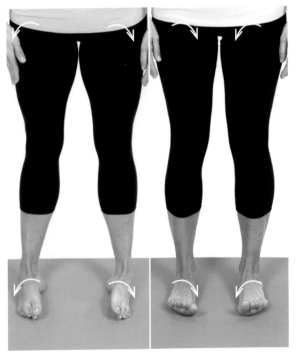

A. Stand with your feet together or hip-distance apart. Shift your weight forward to the front of your feet (as in the left image) and backward toward your heels (as in the right image). Notice how much your head sways forward and backward. When doing Pilates exercises, you want to find the place where your weight is evenly distributed between the front and back of your feet.

B. Roll your weight to the outside of your feet (as in the left image), and then roll your weight to the inside of your feet (as in the right image). Notice how your head stays still but rotation occurs at your hips and pelvis. Again, when doing Pilates exercises, you want to find the place where your weight is evenly distributed between the inside and the outside of your feet.

lower body (knees and hips)

Find Alignment

When doing Pilates exercises, your knees need to stay in alignment with your hips and ankles. However, when straightening your knees, be careful to avoid hyperextending them. If your knees are going into hyperextension, you will notice your legs bow slightly backward. Anyone with knock-knees or bowlegs may find it difficult or even impossible to get into good standing alignment. If this is you, get as close to alignment as possible during the exercises.

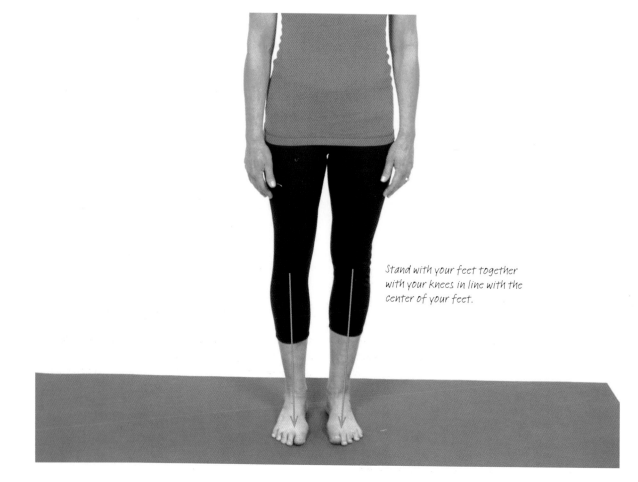

Stand with your feet together with your knees in line with the center of your feet.

Practice Activities

In the following two activities, your knees should stay in alignment with your ankles and hips while moving.

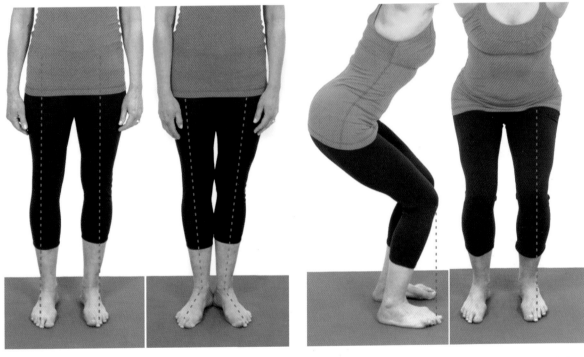

A. Stand with your feet in a parallel position, knees and toes pointed forward (as in the left image). Check that an imaginary line drawn from the centers of your knees would run between your second and third toes. Now rotate your legs out at your hips to come to a turnout position, with your knees and toes facing to the sides (as in the right image). Once again, verify your knees are over the centers of your feet. Good alignment in a parallel or turnout position of your legs helps protect your knees during mat exercises.

B. Squat like you are sitting back in a chair (as in the left image). When squatting, keep your knees behind your toes to avoid putting too much stress on them. Check to make sure your knees are still over the centers of your feet (as in the right image). If you are keeping your foot triangles as described previously, you are helping set a stable base or foundation for good alignment of your knees and hips.

pelvis

Find Alignment

The muscles of your legs, hips, and core attach to your pelvis. Therefore, adjustments in the position of your pelvis not only change how these muscles function, but also change the curves of your lower back. During many Pilates exercises, you want to be in a neutral pelvis position. In a neutral pelvis position, the points on the top-front bones of your pelvis and your pubic bone should be in a level plane.

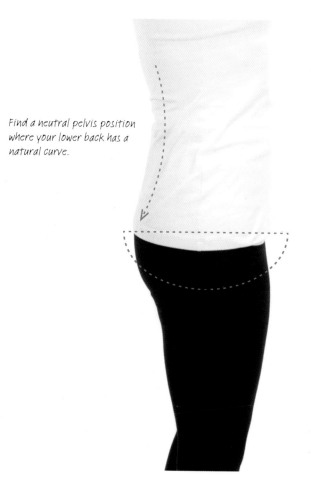

Find a neutral pelvis position where your lower back has a natural curve.

Practice Activities

Think of your pelvis as a bowl filled with water as you try the following activities.

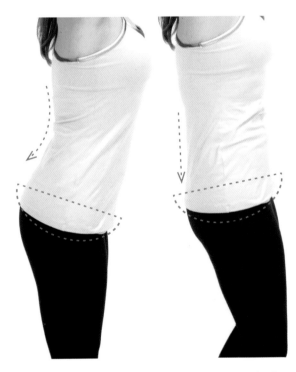

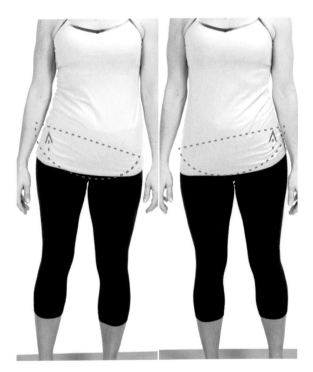

A. Tip the bowl forward, spilling some water onto the floor (as in the left image). Notice when you tip your pelvis forward that your back arches. Next, spill water behind you by tucking your tailbone underneath you, flattening your lower back (as in the right image). Now find the place in between where the water in the bowl is level, which is what you want when doing Pilates exercises.

B. Hike one hip up toward your ribcage, spilling water out of the side of the bowl (as in the left image). Next, hike your other hip up toward your ribcage, spilling water to the other side (as in the right image). Learning where your pelvis is in good alignment in this plane is important when doing side-lying exercises. When lying on your side, you want to avoid these hip hikes.

spine and ribs

Find Alignment

Because so many Pilates exercises involve the spine, Pilates exercises can be highly beneficial when done correctly—and dangerous when done incorrectly. Your ribs attach to the thoracic spine, moving with your spine and expanding with each breath. Therefore, the position of your ribcage is important for upper-body movements, as your ribcage is the foundation for your shoulder blades and arms. Keeping length to your torso and spine during forward and side movements helps support your spine and ribcage.

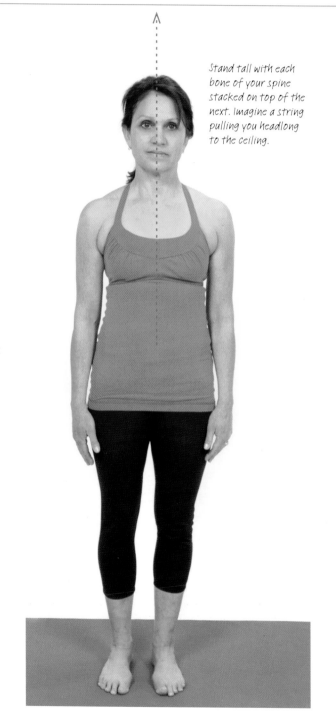

Stand tall with each bone of your spine stacked on top of the next. Imagine a string pulling you headlong to the ceiling.

Practice Activities

If you would like to feel with your hands as you practice these activities for the spine and ribs, place your fingers on the top of your pelvis and a thumb on the bottom of your ribcage.

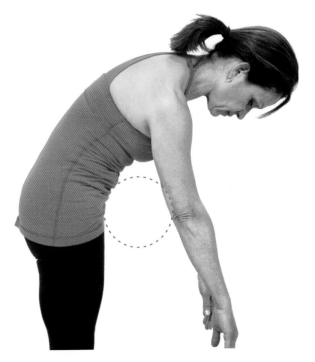

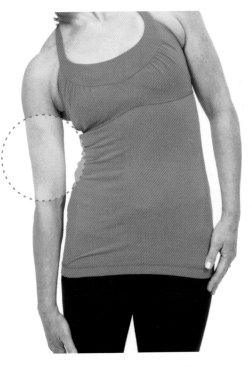

A. Bend forward at your waist, keeping your abdominals relaxed. Notice how the distance from the top of your pelvis and bottom of your ribcage shortens. Now try to lengthen tall by drawing your abdominals in and up (as in the image). Round forward like you are lengthening up and over a big ball. Can you feel how this keeps the space open between the bottom of your ribs and the top of your pelvis? This is the length you want to have during Pilates exercises.

B. Bend to the side, keeping your abdominals relaxed. Notice how your ribcage and pelvis once again move closer together. Now keep your abdominals engaged and lengthen your spine to the ceiling (as in the image). Stretch to the side, keeping the space open from the top of your hips to the bottom of your ribcage, as if rounding up and over a big ball. This length is the desired length you want when doing Pilates motions.

upper body (shoulders and arms)

Find Alignment

Pilates exercises work both the muscles of your arms and the muscles of your back that attach to your shoulder blades. Although the shoulder itself is a ball-and-socket joint, your shoulder blades are triangular-shaped bones found on your back that glide and rotate over your ribcage. During Pilates exercises, you want to keep your shoulders broad and relaxed down instead of lifted up toward your ears.

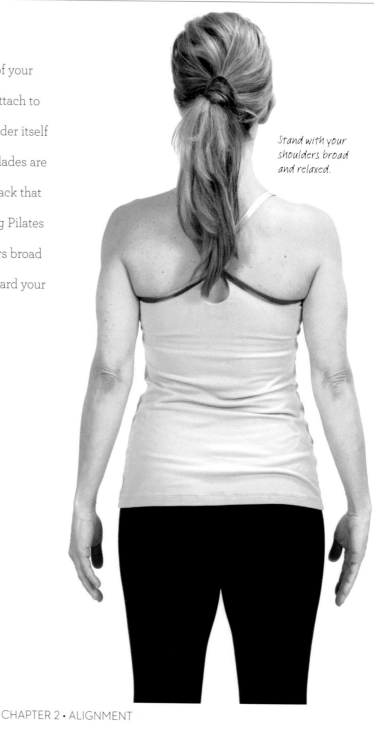

Stand with your shoulders broad and relaxed.

Practice Activities

Imagine your shoulder blades gliding on top of your ribcage as you perform the following movements.

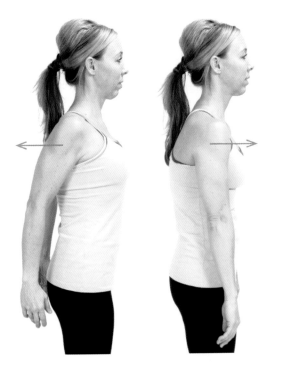

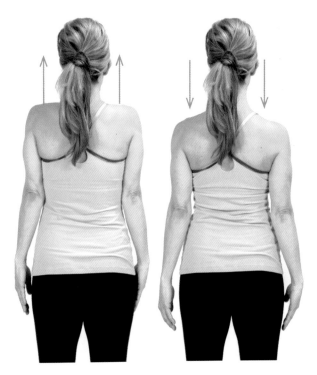

A. Draw your shoulder blades closer to your spine on your back (as in the left image). Notice how the distance between your shoulders gets smaller. Now round your shoulders forward (as in the right image). Once again, the breadth of your shoulder gets smaller. The broadest point in between these two positions is where good alignment is found.

B. Elevate your shoulder blades up toward your ears (as in the left image). Now lower your shoulder blades down to the floor (as in the right image). Feel how too much motion either way creates tension in the muscles of your neck. Find the place where your shoulder blades are resting on your back with your neck relaxed.

head and neck

Find Alignment

When the rest of your body is in alignment, your head should rest directly on top of your shoulders. If you were looking at your head from the side, your neck should stack on top of the rest of your spine and your ears should be in line with your shoulders. Many times, in the poor postures of daily life, your head may drift into a forward posture, which can tighten the muscles of your neck. A subtle change to help keep your head in alignment is to pay attention to where you are looking.

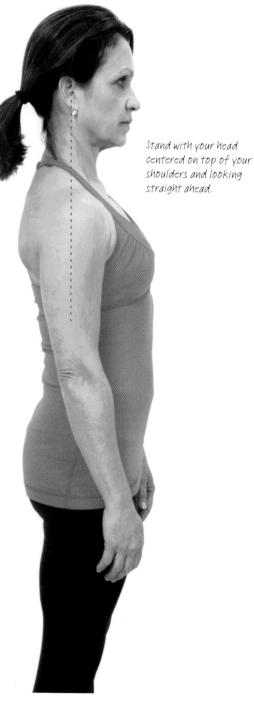

Stand with your head centered on top of your shoulders and looking straight ahead.

Practice Activities

During most Pilates exercises, your head will follow the alignment of the rest of your spine. Try the following alignment exercises to help you understand what to do.

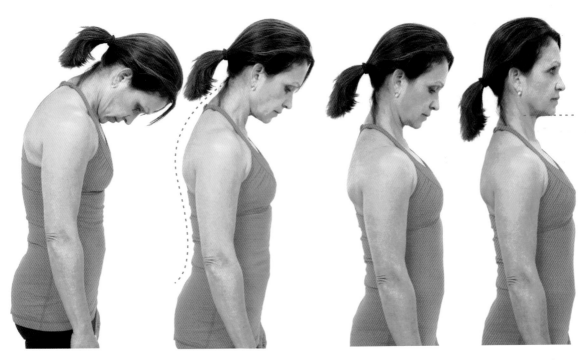

A. Look down toward the floor, bringing your chin down toward your chest as far as you can (as in the left image). This position closes your throat and should be avoided during the Pilates exercises. Now, instead of trying to get your chin close to your chest, imagine a string pulling the back of your head up to the ceiling (as in the right image). Keeping this length helps you avoid collapsing your head too far toward your ribcage. Notice how your upper back also rounds with your neck. Keeping your throat open will help you take care of your neck during your workout.

B. Keeping your neck straight, tuck your chin as if trying to give yourself a double chin (as in the left image). Now find a position where your chin is level to the floor when your mouth is closed (as in the right image). This level position is what should be kept, relative to your spine, during most Pilates exercises.

CHAPTER 3

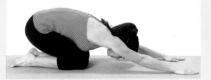

Pilates Essential Practice

Part of Pilates is changing the patterns for how your body moves. In this chapter, you learn simple movements that will prepare you for the exercises later in this book.

These changes require time and practice, so take your time learning the Pilates scoop and breathing in particular, as they will be included in every exercise to come. As Joseph Pilates said in *Return to Life,* "Remember, too, that 'Rome was not built in a day,' and patience and perseverance are vital qualities in the ultimate successful accomplishment of any worthwhile endeavor."

pilates scoop

The navel-to-spine or "scooping" motion of the abdominals is done by your deepest abdominal muscle called the *transverse abdominis*. This muscle wraps around your waist and attaches to your lower back, pelvis, and ribcage. Because it acts as your internal back brace, it is essential to engage it before performing any of the Pilates exercises to help support your spine. The following uses breath to help you find your Pilates scoop.

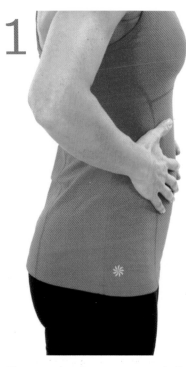

Feel your abdominals draw in and up, as if you're zipping up a tight pair of pants.

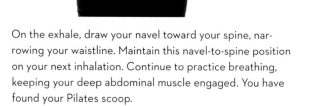

Place your hands on your stomach. Keeping your abdominals relaxed, inhale and allow your stomach to go out.

On the exhale, draw your navel toward your spine, narrowing your waistline. Maintain this navel-to-spine position on your next inhalation. Continue to practice breathing, keeping your deep abdominal muscle engaged. You have found your Pilates scoop.

breathing

During each exercise, breathe with intention and purpose. You should match the breath to your movements, with inhalations through your nose and exhalations out your mouth. If you forget the breathing pattern, continue to breathe at a comfortable pace; however, avoid holding your breath. Learning to breathe deeply while keeping your deep core muscles engaged can take some time to learn, but your lungs, heart, and health will thank you for it.

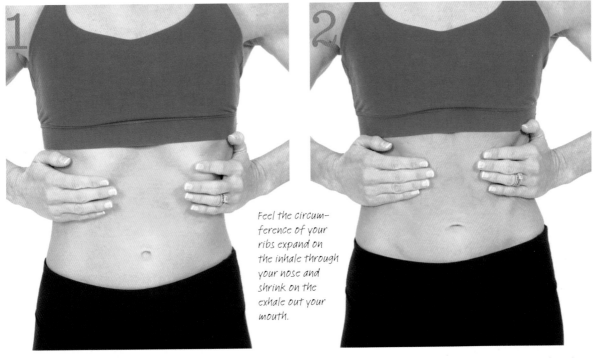

Feel the circum-
ference of your
ribs expand on
the inhale through
your nose and
shrink on the
exhale out your
mouth.

Stand in good alignment with your abdominals scooped. Keep your abdominals engaged as you inhale slowly and deeply through your nose. Feel your ribs expand to the front, back, and sides.

Exhale slowly. Once you have let the air out in a relaxed manner, continue to squeeze the air out of your lungs by using your abdominals. Once you have gotten the extra air out of your lungs, you will feel your ribcage naturally begin the inhalation.

half rolldown

The half rolldown, which is initiated from the curl of your pelvis, teaches you how to come to a C-curve in your spine while keeping the Pilates scoop. Avoid collapsing your spine like you are slouching. Instead, think of coming to a C-shape. This can be done in place of exercises like the roll-up in the next part if you find that too difficult.

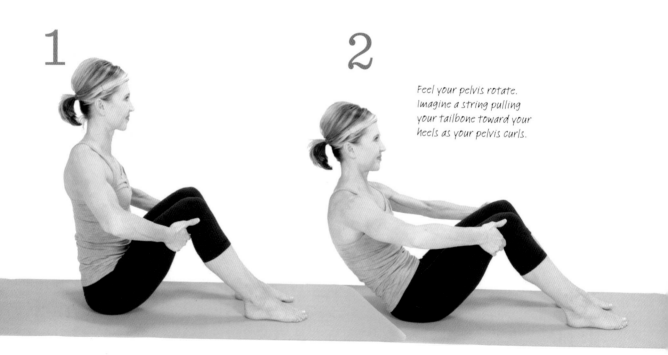

1

2

Feel your pelvis rotate. Imagine a string pulling your tailbone toward your heels as your pelvis curls.

Sit with your feet flat on the floor and your knees bent. Hold onto the back of your thighs with your hands and bring your elbows out to your sides.

Inhale as you curl your tailbone to the front. Let your spine come to a rounded position and roll halfway back. On the exhale, roll up. Once your shoulders are over your hips, turn your pelvis back to the starting position and sit tall. Repeat 10 times.

head, neck, and shoulder lift

Because your head weighs as much as a bowling ball, proper positioning is important to avoid neck tension. Keeping your head, neck, and shoulders lifted is part of several mat exercises you do lying on your back. During the lift, your deep neck and core muscles should help you hold your position. If you ever experience neck tension, do the exercise with your head down on the mat until you're stronger.

1

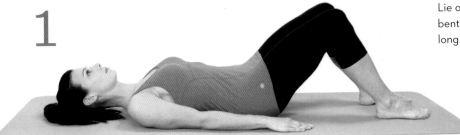

Lie on your back with your knees bent. Inhale as you stretch your arms long toward your toes on the floor.

2

Feel your upper abdominals initiate the head, neck, and shoulder lift.

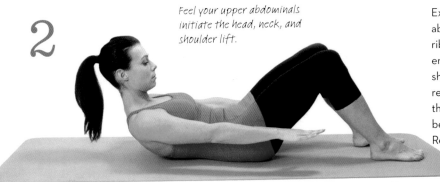

Exhale as you engage your upper abdominals and press your lower ribcage into the floor. With this engagement, lift your head, neck, and shoulders off the mat as your fingers reach long toward your toes. Hold this position, taking several breaths before lowering back to the mat. Repeat 10 times.

pelvic curl

The pelvic curl uses your lower abdominals to rotate your pelvis and lengthen and press your lower back against the mat. To understand this, imagine your pelvis is a bowl open to the ceiling while you are lying on your back. During the pelvic curl, the water will tip out of the bowl toward your face. Awareness of when you are in the pelvic curl is important, as you want to avoid coming to the curl position during mat exercises that require a neutral pelvis.

1

Feel your lower abdominals scoop deeper on the curl.

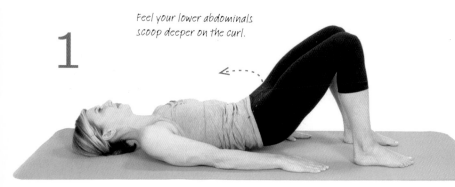

Lie on your back with your feet flat on the floor and your arms at your sides, palms down. Inhale as you curl your tailbone off the mat, lengthening your lower back on the mat. Hold here for several breaths.

2

On an exhale, release the pelvis position and return to a neutral pelvis. Repeat 10 times.

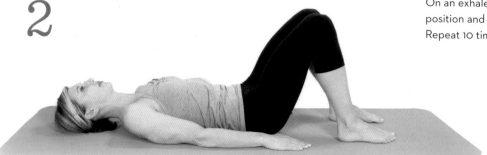

single-leg lift on your back

This exercise teaches you how to move your leg independently of your pelvis and back. Your pelvis should be a neutral position, where the pubic bone and bones at the top of your pelvis are in the same plane parallel to the mat. Make sure you have equal weight on both sides of your pelvis. If you find your pelvis rocks to the side or changes position during the leg lifts, keep practicing and stay patient.

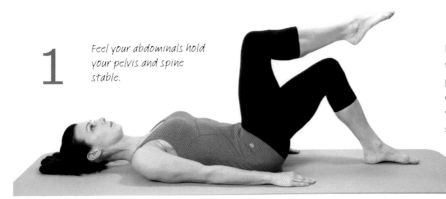

1 *Feel your abdominals hold your pelvis and spine stable.*

Lie on your back with your feet flat on the floor and your arms at your sides, palms down. Inhale as you lift one leg off the floor at a 90-degree angle to your hip and knee. Keep your pelvis stable.

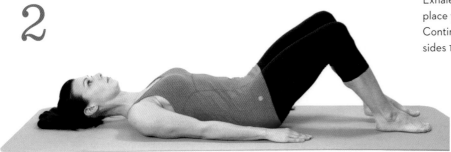

2

Exhale as you lower your leg and place your foot back on the floor. Continue the leg lifts, alternating sides 10 times.

single-leg lift on your stomach

This teaches you how to use your glutes to lift your leg. Before lifting your leg off the floor, lengthen your leg long on the floor, feeling the back of your leg and your gluteal muscles engage. The length helps make sure the right muscles are doing the small leg lift. When ready, lift your leg no more than a few inches off the floor. The goal is not to be able to do a bigger movement, but to use the correct muscles and form to lift.

1

Feel your navel being drawn up and away from the floor throughout the leg lifts.

Lie on your stomach with your legs long on the floor and hip-distance apart. Your hands can be on the mat underneath your forehead, if desired. Inhale as you stretch one leg so long it lifts a few inches off the mat.

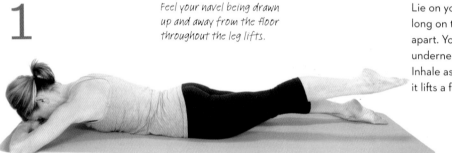

2

Exhale as you lower your leg back to the floor. Continue with small leg lifts, alternating legs 10 times.

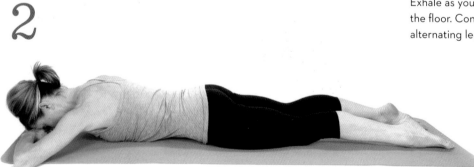

child's pose stretch

This is a delicious stretch for your shoulders, hips, and back and a convenient ending stretch to do after exercises on your stomach. You can come to the child's pose position with a rounded spine or a straight spine. The straight spine focuses the stretch on the muscles of your hips and shoulders, while the rounded spine focuses the stretch on the muscles of your back. If you have knee issues, you can stand and place your hands on a chair to stretch your shoulders and back.

1

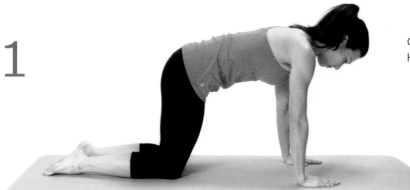

Come to an all-fours position on your hands and knees. Inhale to prepare.

2

Feel the front of your arms, your back, and the back of your hips stretch.

Exhale as you draw your hips toward your heels. Let your body rest against your thighs as you stretch your arms long overhead. Hold for 10 to 30 seconds.

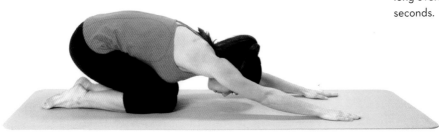

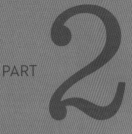

PART 2

Pilates Mat Exercises

Welcome to Pilates mat exercises! In this part, you find a blend of traditional and modern exercises—the only equipment necessary are your mind, your body, and your mat. You may notice the chapters are organized by your body position. The intent is not to do all the exercises in each chapter, but to do a few exercises in each position to work your entire body.

After you've learned these exercises, check out Part 4. There, you'll find routines involving many of the mat exercises. Choose a program based on your comfort level, and start transforming the way you move!

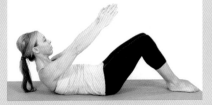

On Your Back

This chapter contains exercises where you lie on, roll on, or bridge your back. Depending on the exercise, your spine will elongate, stabilize, or roll on the mat. Some exercises (such as the hundred or the leg circles) will challenge you to maintain the same back position. Others (such as the roll-up or the double-leg bridge) will have you roll through the spine as you use the mat to feel each bone in your spine articulate one at a time. Your mat will provide you with feedback as to the position of your torso and spine.

hundred

The hundred is a total-body challenge of endurance that activates your cardiovascular system and prepares your body for the rest of the mat exercises. Its name stems from the 100 vigorous arm beats. The corresponding breath pattern of 5 counts of inhalation and 5 counts of exhalation helps you develop breath control. As you perform this, be sure your back is stable and your abdominals are engaged.

BENEFITS

Warms up the body

Strengthens the abdominals

Improves lung capacity

Activates the cardiovascular system

{visualize} bouncing a small ball beneath your hands.

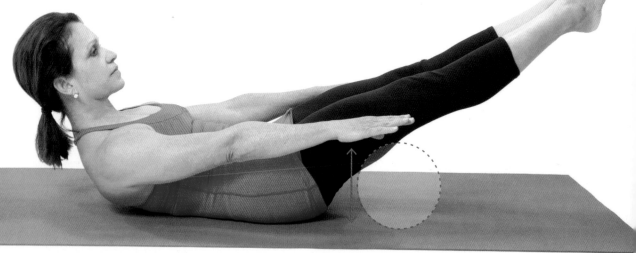

CHAPTER 4 • ON YOUR BACK

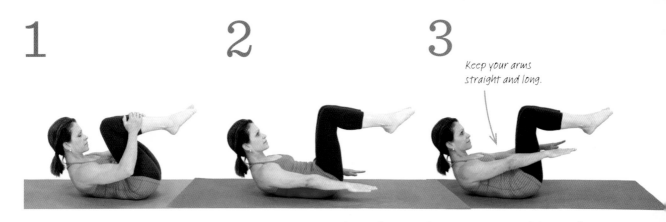

1

Lie on your back with your head, neck, and shoulders lifted and your knees pulled toward your chest.

2

Inhale as you reach your fingers long past your hips. Exhale as you bring your legs out to a 90-degree angle at the hip and knee.

3

Keep your arms straight and long.

Beat your arms up and down 50 beats as if bouncing a small ball under your hands, inhaling for 5 arm beats and exhaling for 5 arm beats.

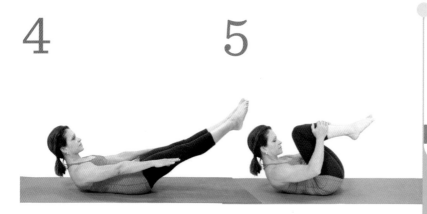

4

Extend your legs at a 45-degree angle and beat your arms up and down 50 more beats, inhaling for 5 arm beats and exhaling for 5 arm beats.

5

Return to starting position by bending your knees toward your chest.

CHALLENGE YOURSELF

Keep your abdominals engaged as you hold your legs at a low angle.

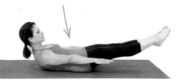

- The lower your legs are to the floor, the greater the abdominal challenge. Hold your feet at eye level throughout the full 100 beats for the greatest challenge.

- Squeeze a ball or ring between your ankles to activate your inner thighs.

roll-up

The roll-up is a challenging exercise for the abdominals. Performing it requires great focus and control, as you can be tempted to use momentum to complete the difficult parts of the exercise. To avoid that, pay careful attention to the way you bring your back off the mat and lower it down.

BENEFITS

Strengthens the abdominals

Develops abdominal control

Teaches spine articulation

{visualize} one bone of your spine rolling up off the mat at a time.

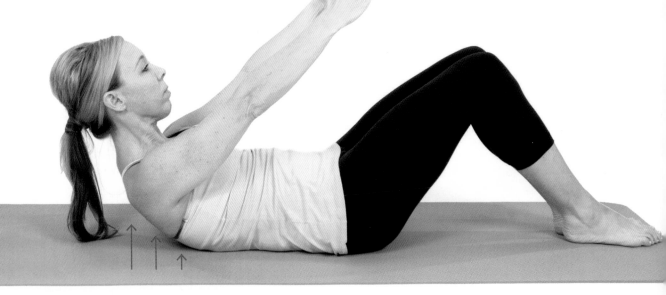

CHAPTER 4 • ON YOUR BACK

1

Lie on your back with your legs slightly bent and your arms resting at the sides of your body.

2

keep your lower ribcage down on the mat to avoid arching your back.

Inhale as you bring your arms over your shoulders to the ceiling. Exhale as you bring your arms overhead.

3

Inhale as you bring your arms toward the ceiling. Exhale to lift your head, neck, and shoulders with your upper abdominals to begin rolling up.

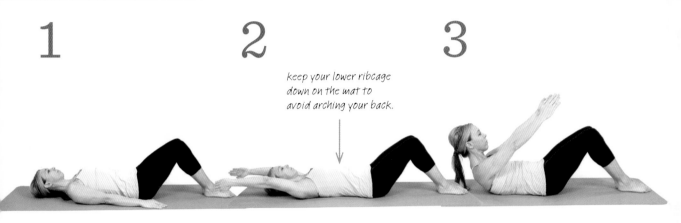

4

Keep your abdominals scooped during the reach forward.

Continue to roll up one bone at a time, taking as many breaths as you need to complete the motion with control.

5

Once you're in a sitting position, inhale to lengthen your spine as you sit tall.

6

Return to a C-curve with your spine by curling at your pelvis to roll down to the mat as you exhale, taking as many breaths as you need to roll down to the mat with control. Repeat the exercise 10 times before returning to starting position.

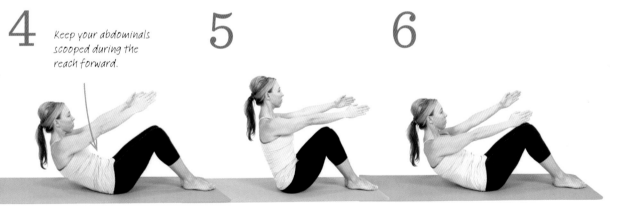

leg circles

Leg circles move your hip in the natural range of the joint. The goal is to stabilize your torso and pelvis by using your core muscles while your leg gracefully moves in a circle. As you do this exercise, work to keep the shape and pace steady in both directions of the circle.

{visualize} your leg as a pencil drawing a steady circle.

1

Bend your legs and place your feet on the mat. Let your hands rest, palms down, at the sides of your body.

2

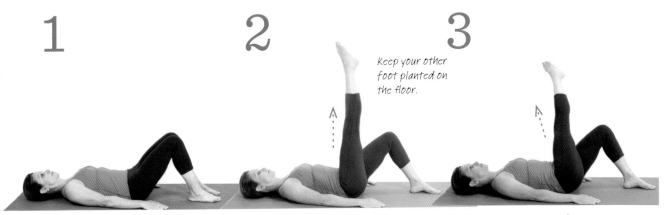

Keep your other foot planted on the floor.

Inhale as you lift one leg off the mat. Exhale as you extend your leg at a 90-degree angle to your body.

3

Inhale as you sweep your leg across your body in a counterclockwise direction, using your core muscles to keep your other leg on the floor and your torso still.

4

On a long exhale, bring your leg down toward the floor at a 45-degree angle.

5

Make sure your pelvis stays stable on the mat.

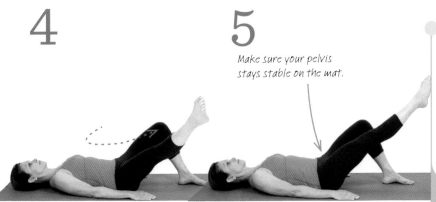

Continue the long exhale as your leg circles out the side and back to a 90-degree angle to complete 1 circle. After 10 circles, reverse the direction of the circle. Repeat with your other leg before returning to starting position.

CHALLENGE YOURSELF

Straighten your nonmoving leg on the mat.

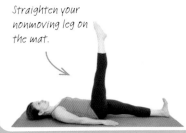

- Straighten your nonmoving leg long on the mat and press your heel into the mat to activate the back of your leg.

- Increase the size of the leg circles to work on your core stability and hips' range of motion.

single-leg stretch

The motions in the single-leg stretch set the foundation for other exercises, such as the double-leg stretch, straight-leg pull, and crisscross. The upper-body lift works your upper abdominals, while the position of your lower body on the mat stretches the back of your hips. While doing this exercise, pay attention to the positioning of your stretching leg by keeping your foot, knee, and hip in line with your shoulder.

{visualize} a continuous line through your shoulder, hip, knee, and ankle.

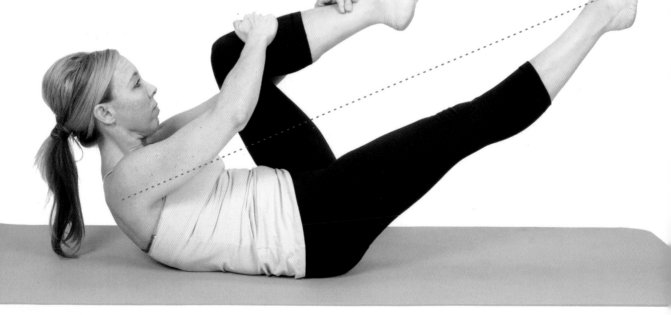

1

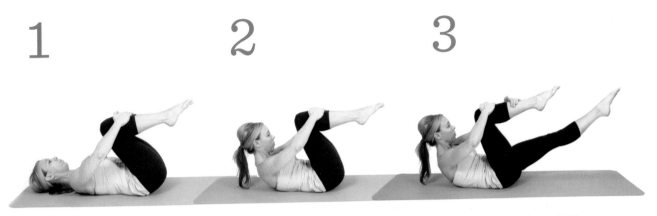

Lie flat on your back on the mat with both your knees to your chest.

2

Inhale as you lift your head, neck, and shoulders and place your hands on the front of your shins just below your knees.

3

Exhale as you extend your left leg at a long, 45-degree angle. Inhale as you pull your right knee toward your chest to begin the exercise.

4

Keep your legs in align-ment with your shoulders.

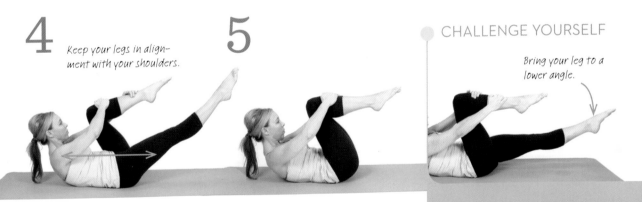

5

Exhale as you switch legs so your left knee is pulled toward your chest and your right knee is extended at a 45-degree angle.

Repeat the exercise, alternating your legs 10 times. Return to starting position by drawing both knees back to your chest.

CHALLENGE YOURSELF

Bring your leg to a lower angle.

- Bring your extended leg to a lower angle until it is eye level for more of an abdominal challenge.

- Perform the exercise at a slower pace to test your endurance.

SINGLE-LEG STRETCH

double-leg stretch

The double-leg stretch follows a similar sequence to the single-leg stretch but requires a greater amount of abdominal strength since both your legs stretch at the same time. To obtain the full benefit of the exercise, your abdominals need to stay engaged with your back on the mat and your abdominals scooped. With practice, you should be able to extend your legs at eye level during the exercise.

BENEFITS

Stretches the hips

Strengthens the abdominals

Develops spine stabilization

{visualize} your navel being pulled deep into the mat as your legs extend.

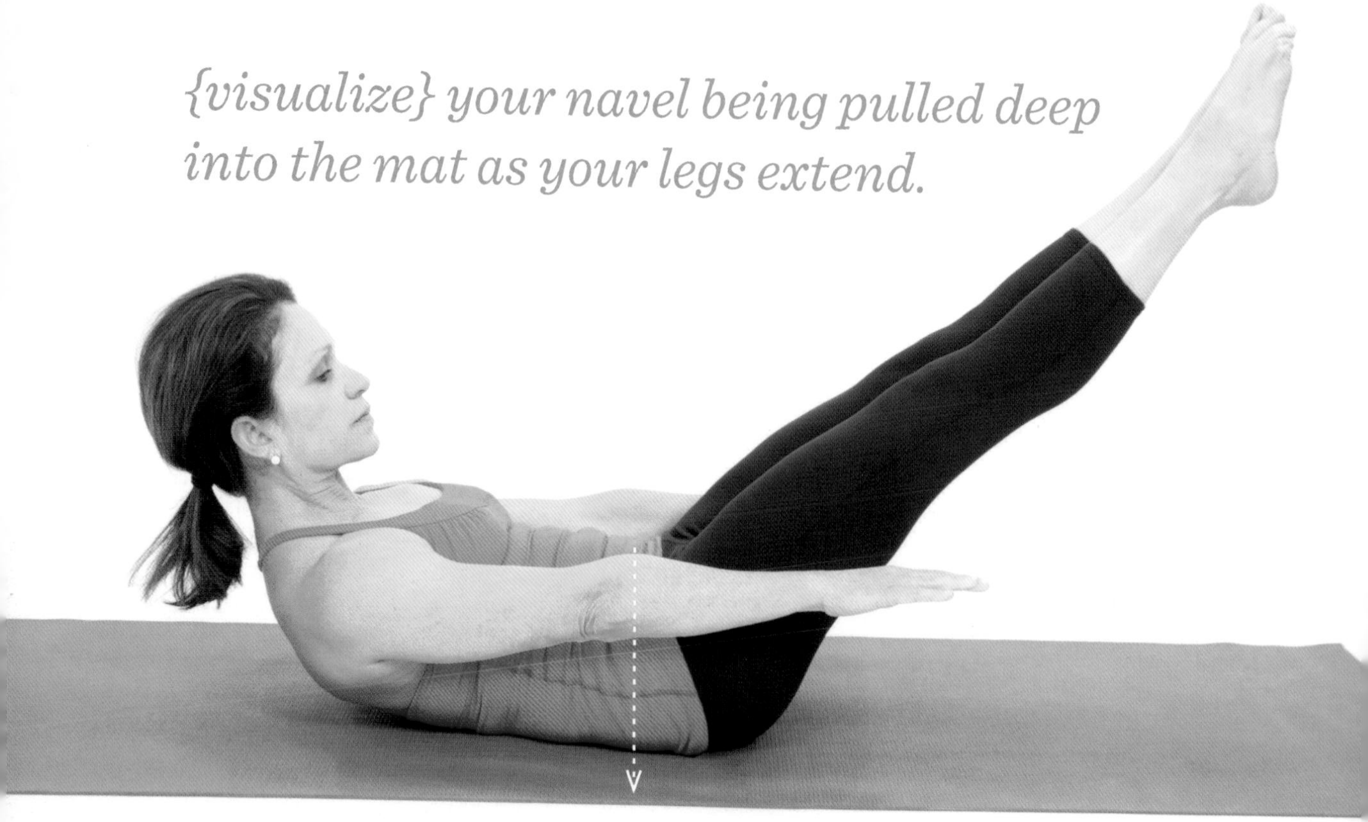

CHAPTER 4 • ON YOUR BACK

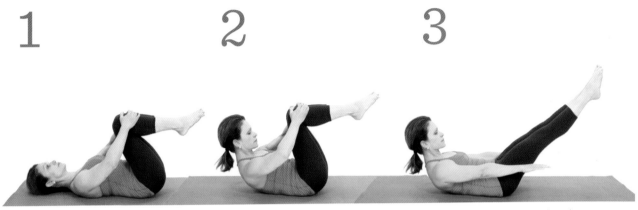

1

Lie flat on your back on the mat. Bend both knees to your chest; lift your head, neck, and shoulders; and place your hands on the front of your shins just below your knees.

2

Inhale as you pull your knees to your chest, keeping your pelvis down on the mat as you do so.

3

Exhale as you extend your legs long at a 45-degree angle and reach your arms long, palms down, at the sides of your body.

4

Inhale as you pull your knees back to your chest. Repeat the exercise 10 times before returning to starting position.

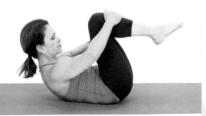

MAKE IT EASIER

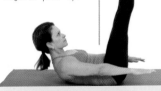

Extend your legs to a 90-degree angle at your hip.

- Bring your legs to a higher angle to the ceiling to lessen your lower abdominal work.
- Leave your head, neck, and shoulders down on the mat to decrease the test to your upper abdominals.

CHALLENGE YOURSELF

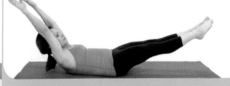

Keep your head, neck, and shoulders lifted as your arms reach overhead.

- Stretch your arms overhead as your legs extend at an angle to increase the challenge to your upper abdominals.
- Bring your legs to a lower angle to focus more attention on your lower abdominals.

DOUBLE-LEG STRETCH

47

straight-leg pull

The straight-leg pull has a similar sequence to the single-leg stretch but provides more of a challenge by keeping your legs straight. This exercise stretches the muscles and tissue along the back of your legs to include your hamstrings. As you perform this, focus on scooping your abdominals deep and keeping your shoulders down and away from your ears as you reach for your legs.

BENEFITS

Strengthens the abdominals

Stretches the back of the legs

Develops spine stabilization

{visualize} your abdominals sinking deeper as you pull your leg toward you.

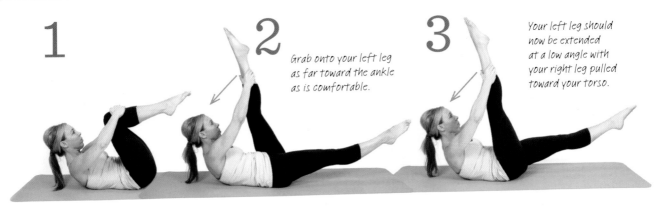

1

2

Grab onto your left leg
as far toward the ankle
as is comfortable.

3

Your left leg should
now be extended
at a low angle with
your right leg pulled
toward your torso.

Bring your knees to your chest and inhale as you lift your head, neck, and shoulders.

Exhale as you extend your left leg over your body toward the ceiling, making sure to keep it straight. Extend your right leg out to a low angle. Inhale as you pull your left leg toward your torso, while you lift your torso toward your leg.

Exhale as you switch the positions of your legs. Inhale as you pull your right leg toward your torso while you lift your torso toward your leg. Repeat the exercise 10 times, alternating legs, before returning to starting position.

● MAKE IT EASIER

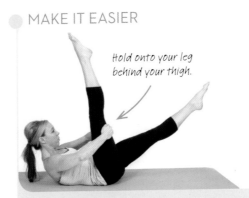

Hold onto your leg
behind your thigh.

- Grab onto your leg behind your thigh or knee for less of a stretch.

- Come to a smaller leg split to decrease the stretch and abdominal challenge.

- Go back to the single-leg stretch to strengthen your abdominals more.

STRAIGHT-LEG PULL

49

crisscross

The crisscross is another abdominal-targeted exercise that, similar to the single-leg stretch, moves the legs in the same alternating pattern. It's important to keep your hip, knee, and ankle in a straight line to avoid sloppy form when performing this. You should also focus on initiating the twist from your oblique abdominals, located along the side of your body, as you move one shoulder toward your opposite hip.

BENEFITS

Strengthens the abdominals

Develops spine stabilization

Teaches coordination

{visualize} one shoulder rotating toward your legs as the other shoulder rotates behind you.

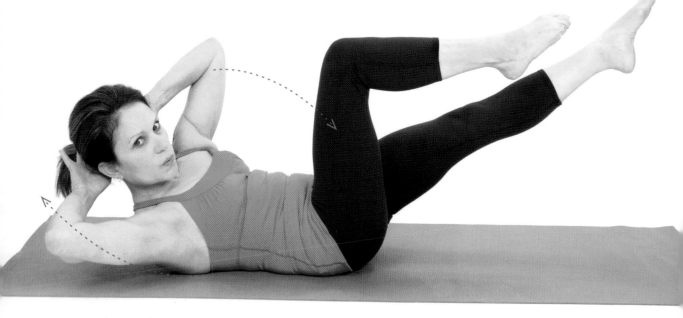

1   2   3

*Your hands are behind your head
to support your head and neck
and to facilitate rotation.*

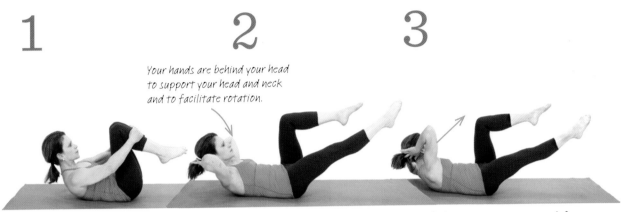

Bring your knees to your chest and lift
your head, neck, and shoulders.

Place your hands behind your head,
with your elbows wide to the side.
Extend your right leg at a 45-degree
angle, and draw your left knee in a
bent position toward your chest.

Inhale as you rotate to your left,
bringing your right shoulder toward
your left hip and knee.

4   5   6

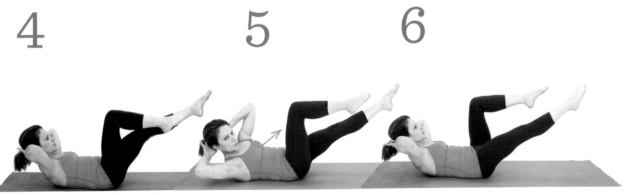

Exhale as you rotate your torso to the
right, extend your left leg 45 degrees,
and draw your right leg toward your
chest in a bent position.

Inhale as you lift your left shoulder
toward your right hip and knee.

Exhale as you rotate your torso to
the left side, extend your right leg
45 degrees, and draw your left
leg toward your chest in a bent
position. Repeat the exercise 10
times, alternating sides, before
returning to starting position.

double-leg lifts

The long lever of your arms and legs in double-leg lifts makes for a great abdominal challenge. The goal of this exercise is to have your head, neck, shoulders, and torso position remain the same as you hinge at your shoulder and hip joints to move your arms and legs. As you do this, only perform the motion in the range you can keep your spine stable on the mat.

BENEFITS

Teaches movement of the shoulders and hips with a stable core

Strengthens the abdominals

Develops spine stabilization

{visualize} your arms and legs coming together and moving apart like a set of double doors opening and closing.

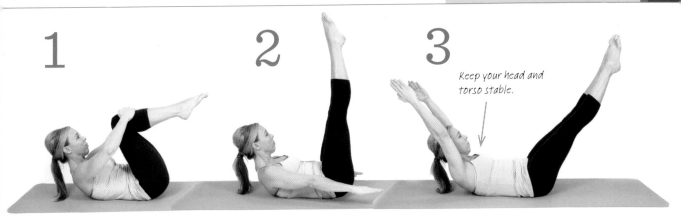

1

Lie flat on your back with both your knees to your chest. Inhale as you lift your head, neck, and shoulders and place your hands on your shins just below your knees.

2

Exhale as you bring your legs up to the ceiling and stretch your arms long at the sides of your body.

3

Keep your head and torso stable.

Inhale as you stretch your arms overhead, keeping your head, neck, and shoulders at the same height, and lower your legs to a 45-degree angle.

4

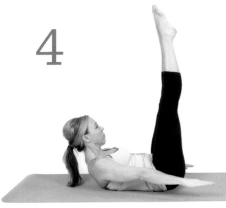

Exhale as you return your legs to a 90-degree angle at the hips and draw your arms down to the sides of your body. Repeat the motion 10 times before returning to starting position.

MAKE IT EASIER

Bring your arms up to the ceiling.

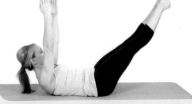

- Perform the exercise with your knees bent at a 90-degree angle for less of an abdominal challenge.
- Bring your arms only to the ceiling for an easier upper-body movement.

CHALLENGE YOURSELF

Gently squeeze the ring between your arms.

- Bring your legs to a lower angle for a greater abdominal challenge.
- Hold a band, ring, or ball between your hands for more of an upper-body test.

DOUBLE-LEG LIFTS

corkscrew

The corkscrew is a great test of oblique control, as you glue your heels together and draw a circle with your legs. The goal is to draw a smooth circle while keeping a steady pace throughout the motion. Start by drawing a small circle the size of a basketball, pressing your heels together to help your legs move as a unit. Once you have perfected small circles, you can increase the size of the circle.

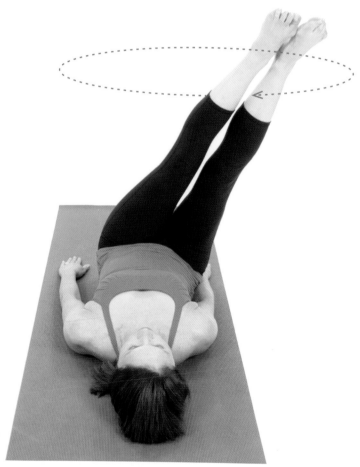

{visualize} your shoulders and rib-cage being glued down to the mat as your legs draw a circle on the ceiling.

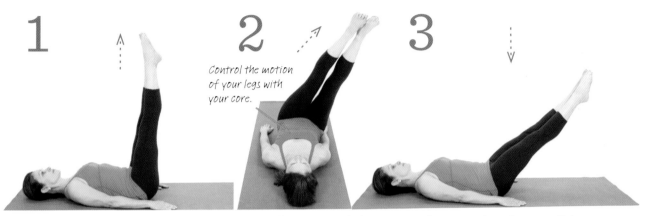

1

Lie on your back with your arms at your sides, palms down. Bring your legs straight up to the ceiling with your heels pressing together.

2

Control the motion of your legs with your core.

Bring your legs to one side, letting the opposite side of your pelvis lift slightly off the mat on the inhale.

3

Lower your legs down at a slight angle, continuing to inhale.

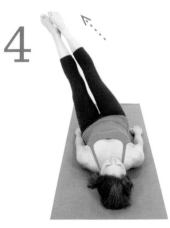

4

Exhale as you start the last half of the circle and your legs come to the other side.

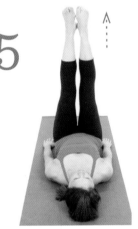

5

Continuing to exhale, sweep your legs back to a 90-degree angle at the hip to complete the circle.

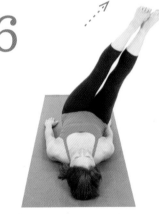

6

After 10 circles in one direction, reverse the direction to draw 10 corkscrews with your feet going the other direction. Draw your knees to your chest to finish.

coordination

This exercise is a great workout for your inner thighs and abdominals—and, like the name states, your coordination. Once in position, your legs open and close quickly as you do a quick exhale. You can think of the different movements like a wave traveling from your head to your legs. Because you have to have a matching breathing pattern, plan on this exercise taking some time to master.

{visualize} your legs opening to a small V-position and quickly closing back together.

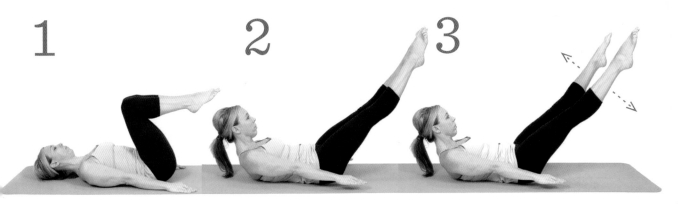

1 Lie on your back with your arms at your sides and your legs bent to your chest.

2 Inhale as you lift your head, neck, and shoulders off the mat. Exhale as you extend your legs long to a 45-degree angle.

3 Inhale as you open your legs to a small V-position.

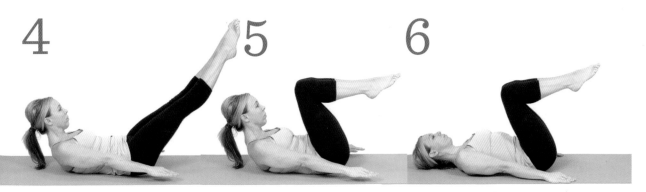

4 Exhale as you quickly draw your legs back together with power and control. Repeat opening your legs on an inhale and closing your legs on a quick exhale 3 times.

5 Inhale as you bend your legs to your chest.

6 Exhale as you lower your head, neck, and shoulders back to the mat. Repeat the exercise 10 times before returning to starting position.

rollover

The rollover develops spine flexibility but requires abdominal strength and control to perform safely. Move only as far as your core can control; otherwise, you may put your body into a position where your abdominals may not be able to support your spine properly. To avoid placing stress on your neck, roll up only until the weight is across your shoulders.

{visualize} one bone of your spine peeling off the mat at a time.

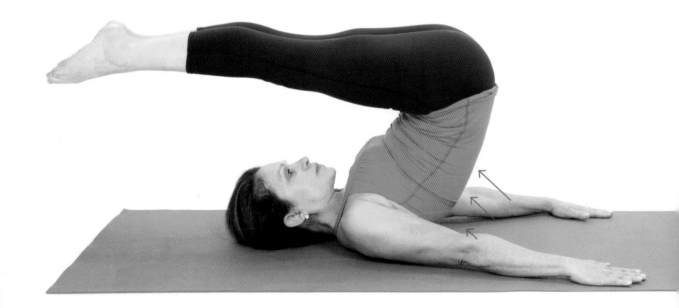

1

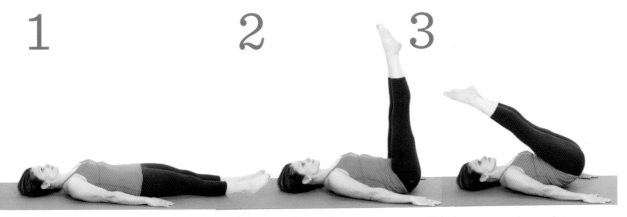

Lie on your back with your arms at the sides of your body, your legs long, and your feet pointed.

2

Inhale as you lift your legs to a 90-degree angle at your hip.

3

Exhale as you continue to bring your legs over your torso, letting your spine come off the mat one bone at a time. Take as many extra breaths as you need to complete the motion.

4

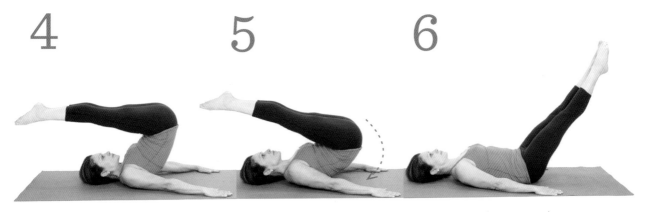

Inhale as you hold the rollover position.

5

Exhale as you begin rolling your spine back down to the mat. Take as many breaths as you need to place your spine back on the mat.

6

Lower your legs to a 45-degree angle as you exhale. Repeat the exercise 5 times before returning to starting position.

jackknife

The jackknife builds off of the motions learned during the rollover and similarly develops spine flexibility and abdominal strength. During this exercise, your legs extend to the ceiling as if doing a handstand with your bodyweight supported across your shoulders. Because this exercise is considered advanced, be sure you have mastered the rollover before trying this.

BENEFITS

Strengthens the back of the arms and hips

Strengthens the abdominals

Teaches spine articulation

Improves flexibility of the spine and hips

{visualize} a hinge at your hips as your legs rotate toward the ceiling.

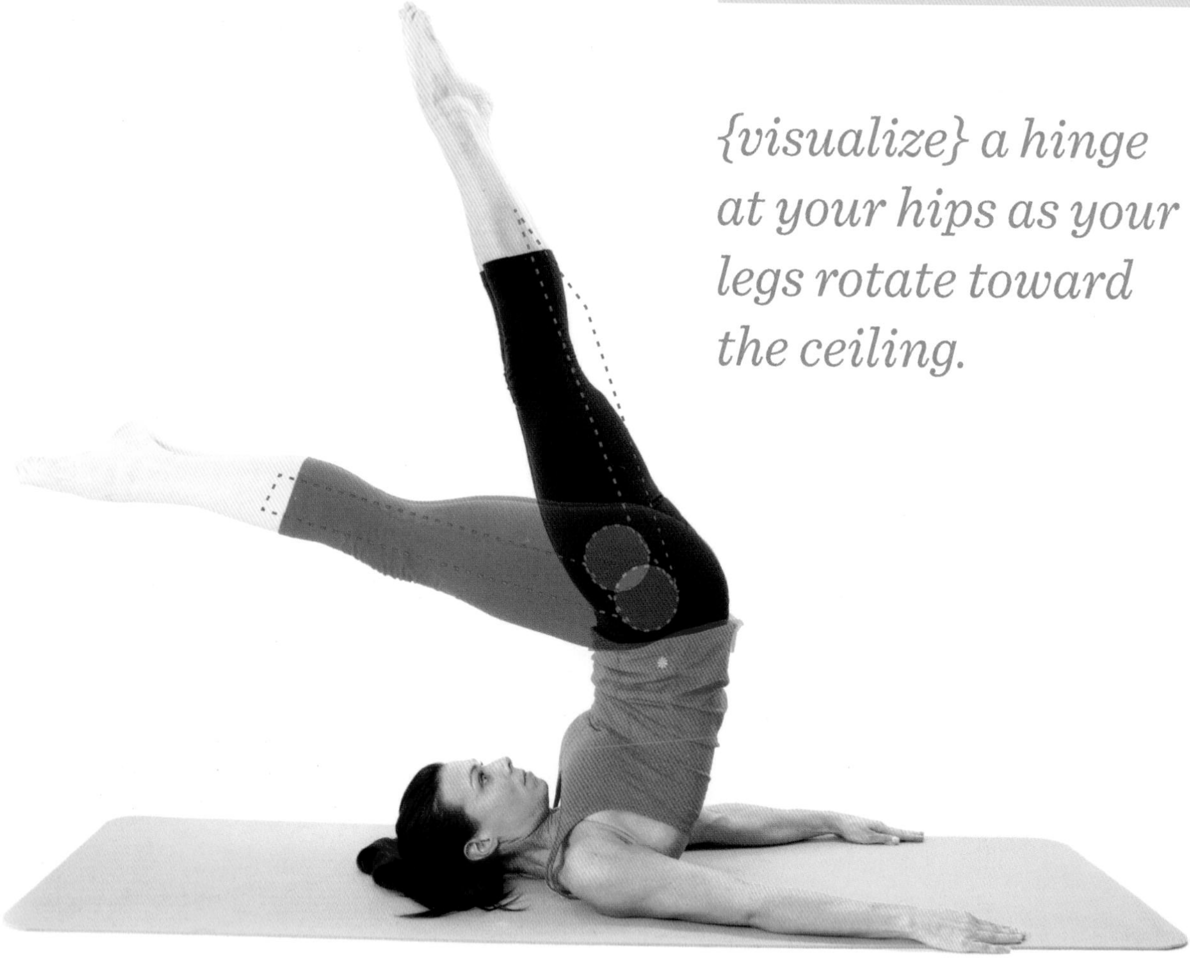

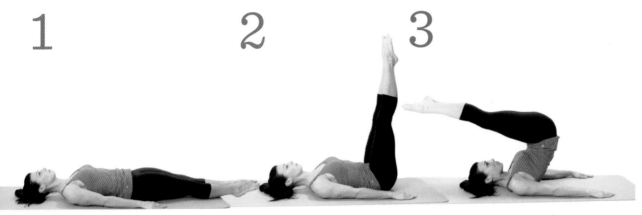

1

Lie on your back with your arms at the sides of your body, your legs long, and your feet pointed.

2

Inhale as you lift your legs to a 90-degree angle at your hip.

3

Exhale as you continue to bring your legs over your torso, letting your spine come off the mat one bone at a time. Take as many extra breaths as you need to complete the motion.

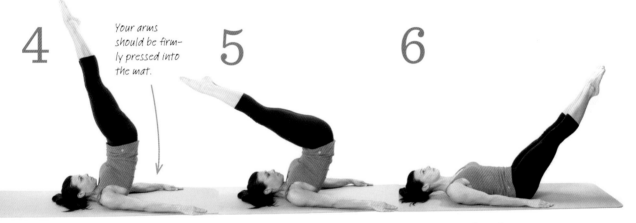

4

Your arms should be firmly pressed into the mat.

Once you are in a rollover position, inhale as you lower your feet to the floor. Exhale as you lift your legs straight up to the ceiling, using your core muscles to keep your pelvis and spine lifted.

5

Inhale as you hold the jackknife position. Exhale as you roll your spine back down to the mat. Take as many breaths as you need to place your spine back on the mat.

6

Lower your legs down to a 45-degree angle as you exhale. Repeat the exercise 5 times. Finish by lowering your legs down to the mat.

neck pull

The neck pull works on developing abdominal control in both a straight hinge and rounded spine. This exercise builds off of the movements learned during the roll-up, with the added challenge of having your hands behind your head for extra resistance. As you perform this, keep your heels pressing into the mat with flexed feet and your elbows wide to the sides.

BENEFITS

Strengthens the abdominals

Develops core control

Teaches spine articulation

{visualize} your spine lengthening straight and long on the hinge back while your elbows stay wide like a butterfly with open wings.

1

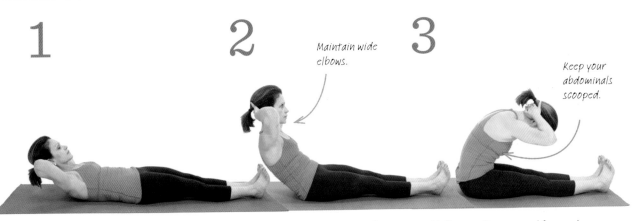

2

Maintain wide elbows.

3

Keep your abdominals scooped.

Lie on your back with your hands behind your head, elbows wide to the sides. Press your heels into the mat and flex your feet. Inhale as you lift your head, neck, and shoulders off the mat.

Exhale as you continue the roll-up, peeling one bone of your spine off the mat at a time.

Roll up until you round forward over your legs.

4

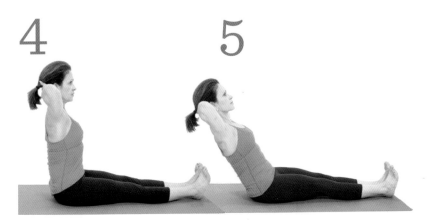

5

Inhale as you roll to a straight spine.

Exhale as you hinge back as far as you can. Curl at your pelvis to come to a rounded spine and roll one bone down to the mat at a time. Repeat the exercise 5 times to finish on your back on the mat.

NECK PULL

teaser prep

The teaser prep works your abdominals and legs and prepares your body for the more-challenging teaser 1 and teaser 2 exercises. In the ideal teaser position, your legs are at a 45-degree angle and your torso is at a matching 45-degree angle in relation to the mat—this "teases" your balance and core. This exercise teaches you a modified version of this ideal position.

BENEFITS

Strengthens the abdominals and legs
Challenges balance
Develops concentration
Teaches control

{visualize} *your arms reaching long at a 45-degree angle parallel to your leg extensions.*

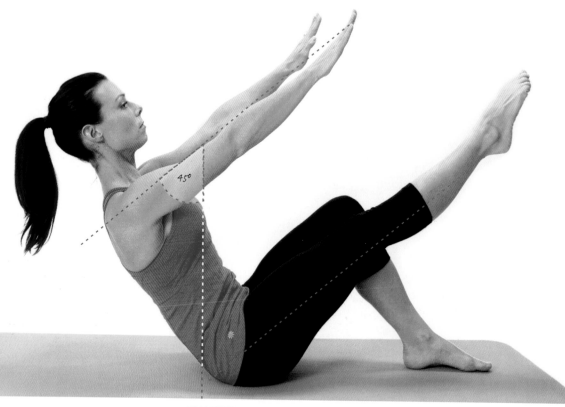

45°

1

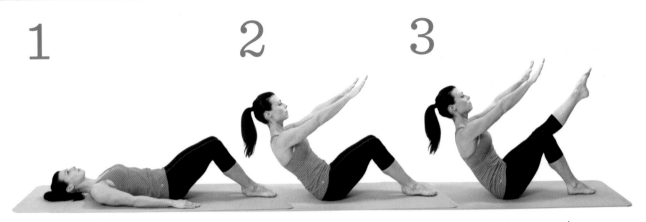

Start on your back with your knees bent and your feet flat on the floor.

2

Inhale as you lift your head, neck, and shoulders. Exhale to roll up to a 45-degree angle with your torso and reach your arms long over your legs.

3

Extend one leg long at a 45-degree angle on an inhale. Exhale as you lower your leg back to the mat.

4

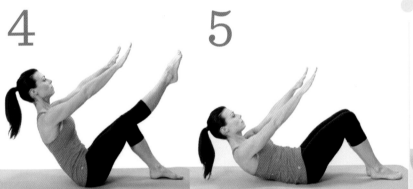

Extend your other leg to a 45-degree angle on an inhale. Exhale as you lower your leg back to the mat.

5

Inhale as you begin the rolldown. Exhale to finish rolling down to the mat. Repeat this series 5 times before returning to starting position.

● MAKE IT EASIER

Do just the torso lift.

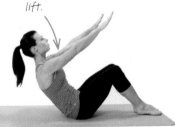

- Keep your knee bent at a 90-degree angle during the leg lift for less of a core challenge.
- Omit the leg extensions and do just the torso lift to simplify the exercise.

teaser 1

This exercise builds off the teaser prep and helps strengthen your legs and abdominals. During teaser 1, you hold your legs at a 45-degree angle as you roll your torso up to a teaser and then down. Be careful to avoid tension in your back while doing the teaser motions. If you experience any back tension, you can either stop or return to the teaser prep to gain more strength.

BENEFITS

Develops concentration

Strengthens the abdominals and legs

Challenges balance

Teaches control

{visualize} your legs holding still and steady at a 45-degree angle throughout.

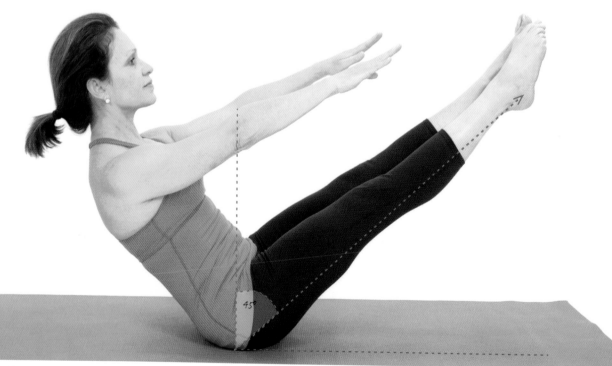

45°

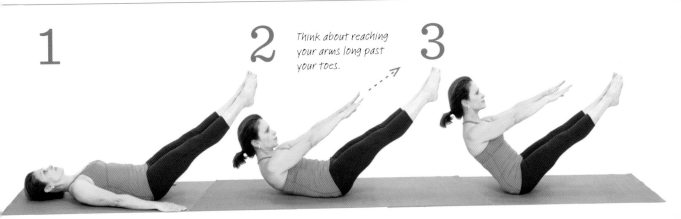

1

Lie on your back with your legs extended long. Lift your legs to a 45-degree angle.

2 *Think about reaching your arms long past your toes.*

Inhale as you lift your head, neck, and shoulders off the mat. Reach your arms long at the angle matching the position of your legs.

3

Exhale as you roll up to a teaser position with your legs and torso each at a 45-degree angle to the mat. Keep your arms reaching in a parallel position over your legs.

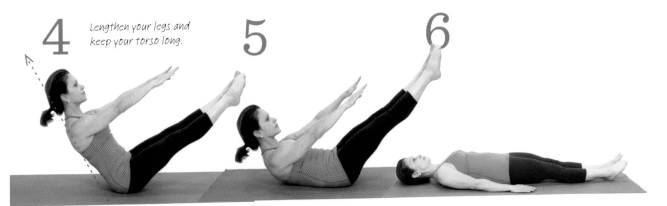

4 *Lengthen your legs and keep your torso long.*

Inhale as you hold the teaser position.

5

Exhale as you turn at your pelvis and roll back down to the mat, keeping your legs at a 45-degree angle throughout. Repeat the motion 5 times.

6

Inhale and exhale as you lower your torso and legs back to the mat to finish.

teaser 2

Like the teaser prep and teaser 1, this really works your abdominals and legs. The teaser 2 requires you to hold a teaser position while lifting and lowering your legs. Once again, be careful to avoid back tension and to keep the work in your core. If you find it too challenging to execute the double-leg lower and lift, consider doing a single-leg lower and lift, alternating your legs as you do so.

{visualize} your arms reaching long past your toes as you hold the teaser position.

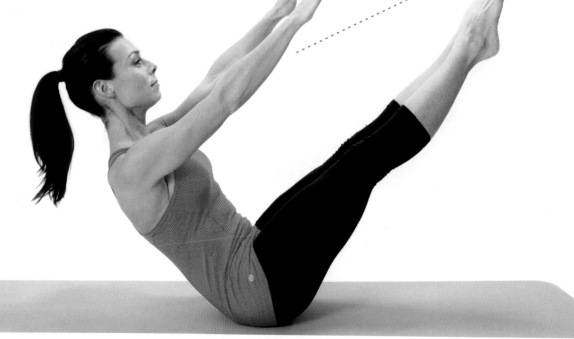

1

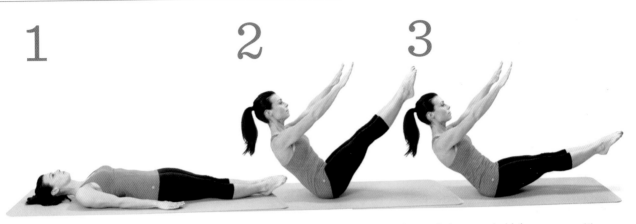

Lie on your back with your back and legs extended long on the mat.

2

Inhale as you lift your head, neck, and shoulders and slightly lift your legs off the floor. Exhale as you continue to lift your legs and torso simultaneously to a teaser position with your torso and legs at a 45-degree angle to the mat.

3

Inhale as you hold the teaser position at the top, keeping your torso steady and lowering your legs toward the mat.

4

Lengthen your legs and keep your torso long.

5

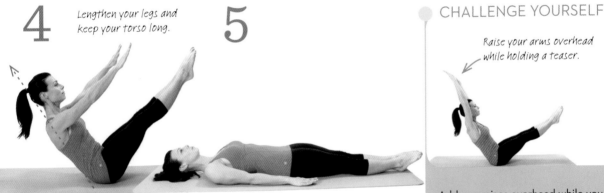

Exhale as you lift your legs back to a 45-degree angle. Repeat the leg lower and lift 5 times.

Inhale and exhale as you roll your torso and lower your legs back down to the mat, returning to starting position.

CHALLENGE YOURSELF

Raise your arms overhead while holding a teaser.

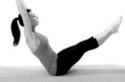

Add arm raises overhead while you hold a teaser position instead of lowering and lifting the legs (also known as teaser 3) for an extra core challenge.

double-leg bridge

Unlike a simple hip lift, the double-leg bridge has you reach your knees long past your toes. This helps keep your torso long and engages your hamstrings and glutes. The ideal position for the bridge portion is your body in a straight line from your knees, the center of your hips, and your shoulders when viewed from the side. The start and end of the bridge is a pelvic curl, which activates your lower abdominals.

BENEFITS

Strengthens the glutes and the muscles on the back of the legs

Develops spine articulation

Lengthens the spine

{visualize} your knees and spine lengthening as you peel your spine off the mat.

CHAPTER 4 • ON YOUR BACK

1

2

3

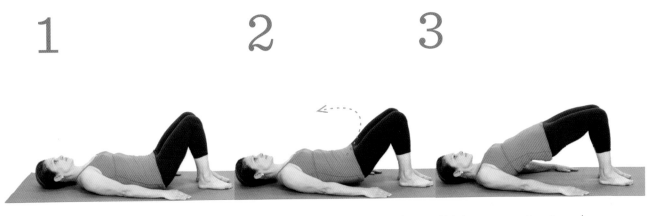

Lie on your back with arms at your sides and your palms down. Place your heels comfortably close to your pelvis.

Inhale as you perform a pelvic curl, pressing your lower back into the mat.

Exhale as you continue to peel one bone of your spine off the mat until you're in a bridge position with your bodyweight supported across your shoulders.

4

5

CHALLENGE YOURSELF

Gently squeeze the ball while holding your heels high off the mat.

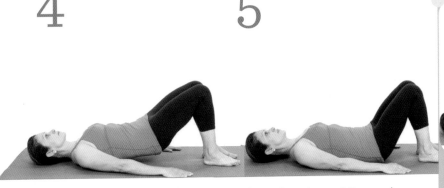

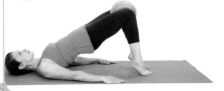

Inhale and exhale as you slowly roll back down to the mat.

Release the pelvic curl. Repeat the bridge 10 times before returning to starting position.

- Hold a ball between your knees for more inner-thigh and pelvic floor work.
- Lift your heels off the ground to work your calves and come to a higher lift during the bridge.

DOUBLE-LEG BRIDGE

single-leg bridge kicks

Unilateral exercises like the single-leg bridge kicks help bring balance to your body. This is step up from the double-leg bridge, so make sure you're proficient at that first before attempting this exercise. When performing this exercise, stay focused on keeping your pelvis stable and level as you lift one leg for a kick—this stability helps strengthen your glutes and legs.

{visualize} your knees and spine lengthening as you peel your spine off the mat.

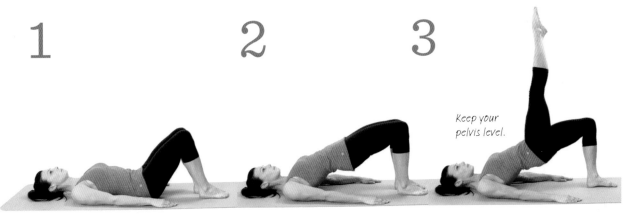

1

Lie on your back with your arms at your sides, palms down. Place your heels comfortably close to your pelvis, keeping your feet flat on the floor.

2

Inhale as you perform a pelvic curl, pressing your lower back into the mat. Exhale as you continue to peel one bone of your spine off the mat until you're up in a bridge position.

3

Keep your pelvis level.

Inhale as you lift one leg up to the ceiling, making sure your hips don't drop down to the mat.

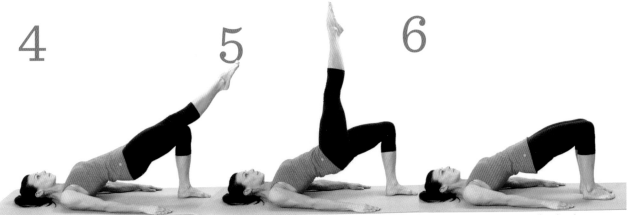

4

Exhale as you lower your leg toward the floor until it reaches your other knee.

5

Inhale as your lift your leg back up to the ceiling.

6

Exhale as you place your leg back down on the floor. Repeat the exercise 10 times, alternating legs. Place your leg back on the mat and roll down to return to starting position.

SINGLE-LEG BRIDGE KICKS

rolling like a ball

Rolling like a ball requires balance and core control to maintain the same body position as you roll. To do this exercise, you need enough abdominal strength to hold a steady C-curve. As you perform it, make sure to roll at a steady pace only until the weight of your body is between your shoulder blades—this helps you avoid stressing your neck.

{visualize} your body as a ball rolling halfway back, pausing, and reversing.

1

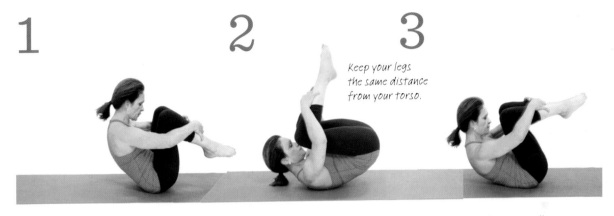

Sit with your knees bent to your chest. Have your spine rounded in a deep C-shape. Look at the top of your knees.

2

Keep your legs the same distance from your torso.

Inhale as you roll back, maintaining the same body position.

3

Exhale as you begin to roll up.

4

Your feet will be off the floor while you balance on the back of your pelvis.

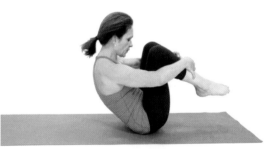

Continue exhaling as you roll up to balance in a sitting position, keeping your feet off the floor the entire time. Repeat the exercise 10 times.

● MAKE IT EASIER

Practice lengthening and rounding your spine.

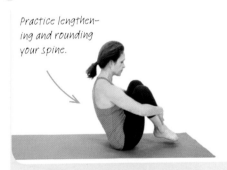

- Hold the rolling-like-a-ball position and breathe in the deep C-curve without rolling for less of a balance challenge.

- Hold the rolling-like-a-ball position and practice lengthening and rounding your spine to improve your core control.

ROLLING LIKE A BALL

75

open-leg rocker

In the open-leg rocker, you perform a roll while your legs are in a V-position. This more-challenging exercise requires lower-body flexibility and greater abdominal control to balance after each roll, so make sure you've mastered rolling like a ball before trying this. Also, as with rolling like a ball, protect your neck by rolling only until your weight is between your shoulder blades.

BENEFITS

Stretches the back of the legs

Massages the back and spine

Challenges balance

Improves core control

{visualize} a tall C-curve to your spine.

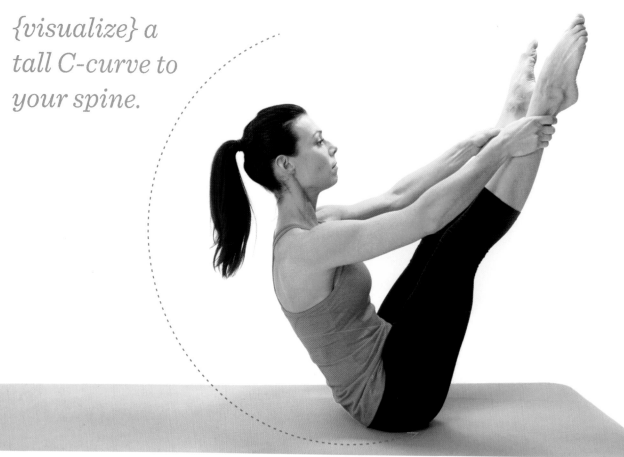

1

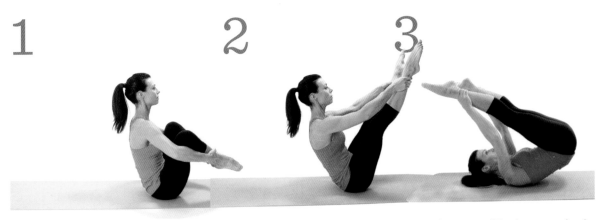

Sit with your knees bent to your chest with your feet off the mat while you balance on the back of your pelvis. Round your spine to a deep C-shape.

2

Inhale as you open your legs to the starting position, with your legs in a V-position. Hold onto your legs near your ankles.

3

Exhale as you roll back to your shoulder blades.

4

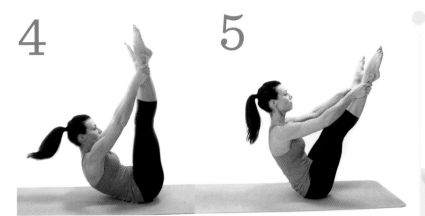

Inhale as you begin to roll up.

5

Continue the inhale as you roll back to sitting and balance at the top. Repeat the rollback 10 times before returning to starting position.

● MAKE IT EASIER

Make sure to round your spine.

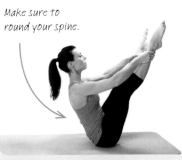

- Hold the open-leg rocker position without rolling to practice your core control.
- Keep your legs slightly bent during your rolls for less of a stretch to the back of your legs.

seal

The seal is a more-advanced form of rolling like a ball in which your legs are drawn closer to your body, requiring good balance. In this exercise, your heels beat together twice at the top of the motion and again at the end of the rollback. When I have taught this exercise to preteen students, we have enjoyed adding a quick "arf, arf" like a seal to each of the heel beats.

BENEFITS

Massages the back and spine

Improves core control

Challenges balance

Develops coordination

{visualize} your heels beating like a seal's flippers.

1

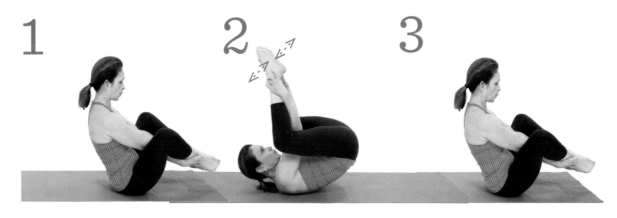

Bring your legs to your body with your spine rounded and your arms inside your legs. With your knees wide to the side, grab under your ankles on the sides closest to the mat. Inhale as you hold the seal position.

2

Exhale as you roll back. Pause when you are back and beat your heels together twice.

3

Inhale as you roll your spine back to a sitting position, balancing without allowing your feet to touch the mat.

4

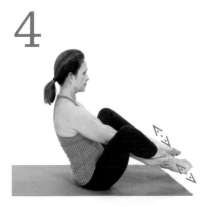

Beat your heels together twice. Repeat the exercise 10 times.

● MAKE IT EASIER

Beat your heels together.

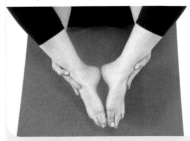

- Hold the seal position while practicing the heel beats without rolling for less of a test to your balance.

- Practice rolling like a ball for a less-challenging leg position.

SEAL

single-side leg lower and lift

During the single-side leg lower and lift, your hips and pelvis roll with abdominal control. How far you stretch your leg to the side is determined by how flexible your inner thighs are. The rotation should occur with just the lower body, while your upper body and shoulders stay down on the mat. Even though you are alternating which leg is held vertically, one of your legs should always be lifting vertically to the ceiling.

BENEFITS

Develops core control

Stretches the inner thighs and legs

Improves spine rotation

{visualize} your moving leg lowering directly to the side.

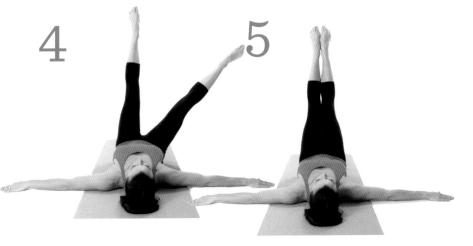

1 Lie on your back with your legs straight and at a 90-degree angle to your hips. Place your arms out in a T-position with your palms down. Press your arms into the floor and anchor your shoulder blades to the mat.

2 Inhale as you lower your left leg straight to the side, making sure it lowers directly to the side instead of at an angle. Keep your right leg up toward the ceiling as the right side of your pelvis rolls slightly off the mat.

3 Exhale as you draw your right hip back to the mat and lift your left leg back up toward the ceiling.

4 Inhale as you lower your right leg straight to the side. Keep your left leg up toward the ceiling as the left side of your pelvis rolls slightly off the mat.

5 Exhale as you draw your left hip back to the mat and lift your right leg back up toward the ceiling. Repeat the exercise 10 times, alternating sides.

double-side leg lower and lift

The double-side leg lower and lift adds a few more steps to the single-side leg lower and lift—as both your legs go to the side, there is a long stretch along the side of your body and your top leg. You may want to hold the rotation stretch, feeling a long line from the tips of your toes to your opposite hand on the floor, to work on your flexibility.

{visualize} your upper body and shoulders being glued to the mat.

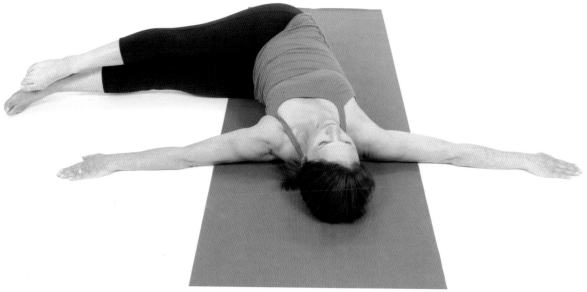

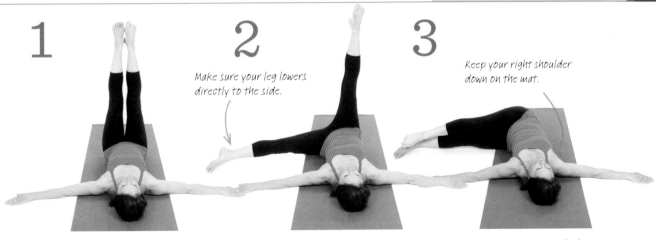

1

2

Make sure your leg lowers directly to the side.

3

Keep your right shoulder down on the mat.

Lie on your back with your legs straight and at a 90-degree angle to your hips. Place your arms out in a T-position with your palms down. Press your arms into the floor and anchor your shoulder blades to the mat.

Inhale as you lower your left leg straight to the left side on the floor. Keep your right leg up toward the ceiling for as long as it can, letting the right side of your pelvis roll off the mat.

Exhale as you lower your right leg directly on top of your left leg. Reach your right leg long while you reach your right arm long in the opposite direction for a deep rotation stretch.

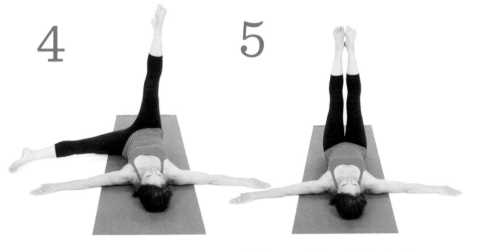

4

5

Inhale as you lift your right leg back up toward the ceiling, using your core to roll your pelvis.

Exhale as you lift your left leg back toward the ceiling. Repeat the side leg lower and lift to the other side. Repeat the exercise 10 times, alternating sides.

CHAPTER 5

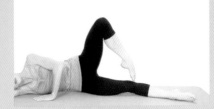

On Your Side

This chapter is all about doing leg work on your side. Your gluteal muscles and the muscles of your hips and pelvis—which are strengthened with these exercises—are important for balance, standing, and walking. You will find that all of the exercises except for one (kneeling side kicks) can be done either with your torso flat on the mat, head lifted, or with your torso lifted and supported by your elbow. The former is an easy position; however, with the latter position, you must be careful to keep your shoulder down and away from your ear and your ribcage lifted away from the floor (in other words, avoid letting your side slouch to the floor).

leg lift and lower

The side-lying leg lifts in this exercise are great for strengthening your glutes and hip. They can be done either with your leg in a parallel position with your knee facing forward or in a turnout with your leg rotated to the ceiling. If you're looking for a larger range of motion, go with the turnout, which opens your hip joint. To perform this exercise properly, focus on keeping your core and pelvis stable.

{visualize} your shoulders and hips being stacked vertically.

1

Your top hand can rest on the floor in front of you.

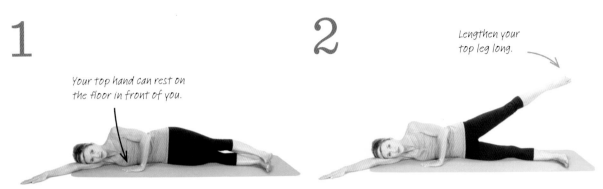

Lie on your side with your back straight, as if it's up against a wall. Bring your legs straight and about a foot in front of your body, with your top leg in a parallel or turnout position.

2

Lengthen your top leg long.

Inhale as you lift your top leg up to the ceiling with a pointed foot.

3

Lead the leg lower with your heel.

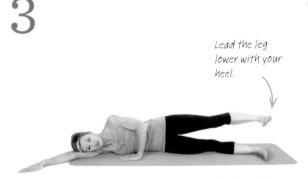

Exhale as you press your leg back down with a flexed foot, imagining it moving as if in a swimming pool. Repeat the exercise 10 times on one side, and turn over to the other side and do the exercise again. Return to starting position.

CHALLENGE YOURSELF

Keep your shoulders down.

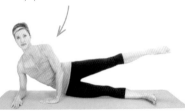

- Repeat the leg lifts, reversing the flex and point motions, for a second set of the exercise.

- Make your leg motion larger to work on your hips' range of motion.

- Come up on your elbow for a more-challenging torso and core position.

front and back sweeps

During the front and back sweeps, your hip flexors and glutes get a good workout as you bring your leg to the front and sweep it to the back respectively. When doing this exercise, avoid letting your torso rock to the front or back. Move with precision, keeping your leg lifted at the same height and parallel to the floor throughout all the sweeps.

BENEFITS

Strengthens the glutes

Teaches hip flexor and glute control

Develops core stabilization

{visualize} your leg moving in a plane parallel to the floor.

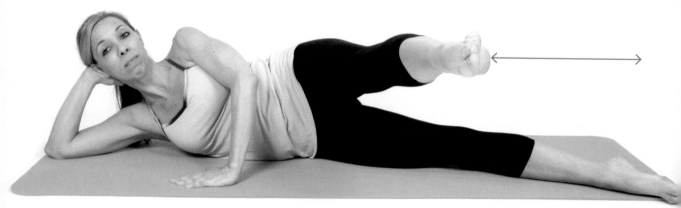

1

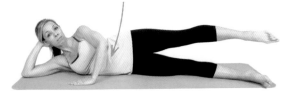

Allow your top hand to rest on the floor in front of you, if you'd like.

Lie on your side with your back straight, as if it's up against a wall. Bring your legs straight and about a foot in front of your body, with your top leg in a parallel position. Bring your top leg to a horizontal position in line with your hip joint.

2

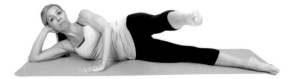

Inhale as you sweep your leg to the front with a pointed foot, only sweeping as far as you can keep your pelvis, torso, and upper body still.

3

Don't arch your back; keep your ab-dominals engaged.

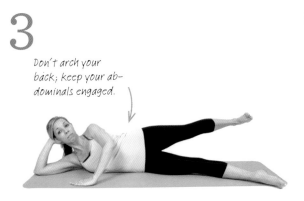

Exhale as you bring your leg through the center to the back with a flexed foot, keeping the sweep motion small. Repeat the exercise 10 times on one side, and turn over to the other side and do the exercise again.

CHALLENGE YOURSELF

Come up on your elbow with your top arm toward the ceiling.

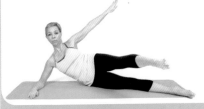

- Make your leg sweeps larger to work on your range of motion.
- Come up on your elbow for a more-challenging torso and core position.
- Take your top arm up to the ceiling to challenge your core and balance.
- Repeat reversing the flex and point motion for a second set.

side-lying leg circles

Side-lying leg circles are great exercise for your hips. To start, keep your leg circles small—about the size of a basketball. Once you can do small circles while keeping your core stable, gradually increase the size of the circle. To work on your hips' range of motion, let your leg come to a rotated position as you take it up to the ceiling and return to a parallel position as your leg circles near the floor.

BENEFITS

Strengthens the muscles of the hips

Lubricates the hip joints

Improves the hips' range of motion

Develops core stabilization

{visualize} your back and pelvis staying stable, as if up against a wall, during each circle.

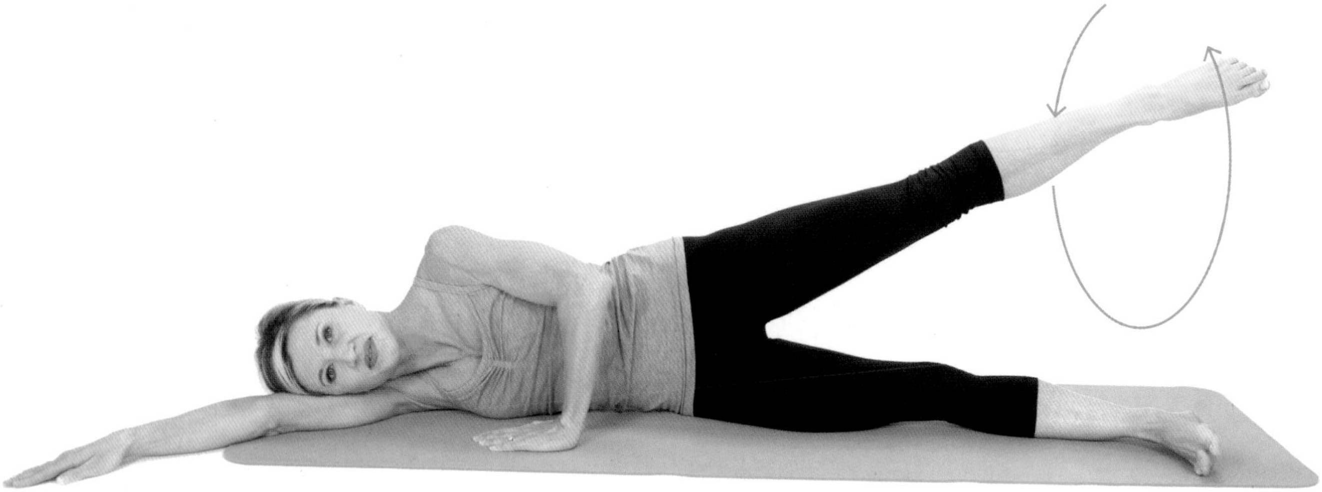

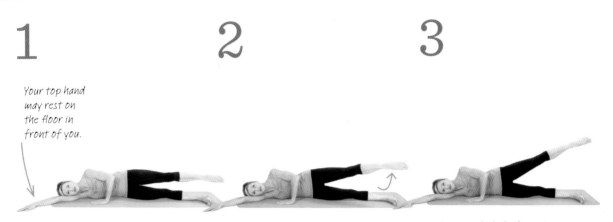

1

Your top hand may rest on the floor in front of you.

Lie on your side with your back straight, as if it's up against a wall. Bring your legs straight and about a foot in front of your body. Lift your top leg to a horizontal position in line with your hip.

2

Inhale as you sweep your leg to the front and up in an arc.

3

Finish your inhale by bringing your leg up at the top of the circular motion.

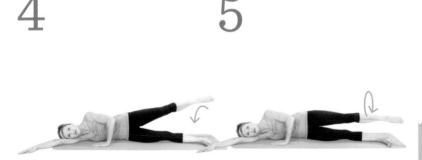

4

Exhale as you lower your leg down and to the back.

5

Finish the exhale as you lower your leg down and to the front, repeating the circle 10 times. Once you have repeated the circle this direction, repeat the circle the other direction. Repeat the exercise with your other leg.

● CHALLENGE YOURSELF

Come up on your elbow with your top arm toward the ceiling.

- Come up on your elbow for a more-challenging torso and core position.
- Take your top arm up to the ceiling for a greater test of your core and balance.

SIDE-LYING LEG CIRCLES

side-lying bicycles

During the side-lying bicycles, your top leg makes a motion like pedaling a bicycle while remaining in a parallel position throughout the exercise. As you pedal both forward and backward, pay attention to the stability of your pelvis as your knee bends and straightens.

BENEFITS

Strengthens the muscles of the hips
Teaches hip flexor and glute control
Develops core stabilization

{visualize} your leg moving a large pedal.

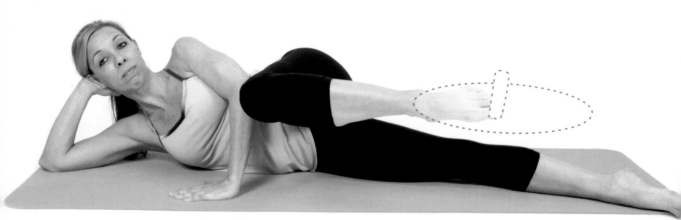

1

Feel free to rest your top hand on the floor.

Lie on your side with your back straight, as if it's up against a wall. Bring your legs straight and about a foot in front of your body. Lift your top leg to a horizontal position in line with your hip.

2

Inhale as you sweep your leg to the front.

3

Continue the inhale as you bend your knee at a 90-degree angle.

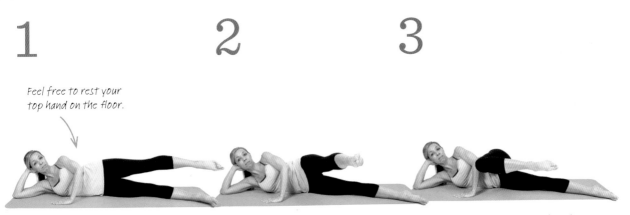

4

Keeping your knee bent at a 90-degree angle, move your entire leg to the back, slightly behind your body.

5

Exhale as you straighten your leg behind your body.

6

Repeat by inhaling and sweeping your leg to the front. Perform the bicycle motion 10 times before reversing the direction to pedal backward. Repeat the exercise with your other leg.

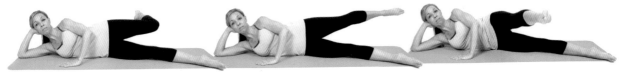

SIDE-LYING BICYCLES

side-lying leg develope

The side-lying leg develope is a similar motion to the side-lying bicycle, except your leg is held in a turnout position throughout. This change in position helps work your hip rotators. As you perform this exercise, the toe of your top leg gently slides along your bottom leg until it reaches your knee.

BENEFITS

Improves hip rotation and flexibility

Strengthens the muscles of the hips

Develops core stabilization

{visualize} your leg stretching long, like the leg of a dancer.

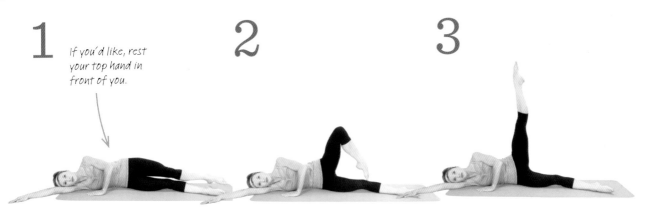

1
If you'd like, rest your top hand in front of you.

Lie on your side with your back straight, as if it's up against a wall. Bring your legs straight and about a foot in front of your body, with your top leg in a turnout position.

2
Inhale as you begin bending your top leg. Let your toe follow the inside of your bottom leg until it reaches your knee.

3
Exhale as you extend your leg up to the ceiling with a pointed foot.

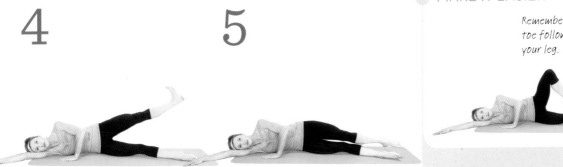

4
Continue with the exhale as you flex your foot and lower your leg back down.

5
Point your foot to return to starting position. Repeat the exercise 10 times before reversing. When you reverse, inhale as you lift your leg to the ceiling and exhale as you bring your toe to your knee. Straighten your knee back to starting position.

MAKE IT EASIER

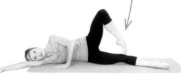

Remember to let your toe follow the inside of your leg.

- Perform just the motion of bringing your toe as far up to your knee as you are able to practice only the easiest part of the exercise.

- Try doing the side-lying leg lifts in a turnout position to practice part of the exercise until you are ready for the full exercise.

SIDE-LYING LEG DEVELOPE

inner thigh lifts

The inner thigh lift is a great way to strengthen your inner thigh muscles. Keep your lift small during this exercise by lifting your leg no more than a few inches off the floor. Because your top leg is bent up to the front, you may feel a stretch in the back of your top hip if your hips are tight. Use the starting position as an opportunity to stretch your hip.

{visualize} your bottom leg lengthening so long it slightly lifts off the floor.

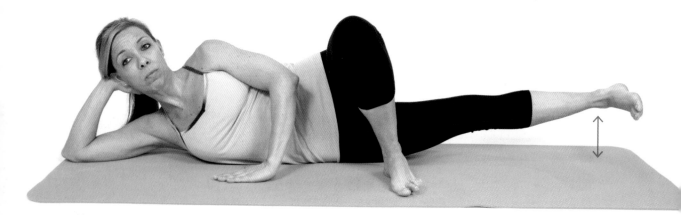

1

Your top hand may rest on the floor in front of you.

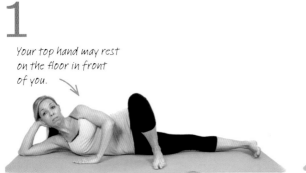

Lie on your side with your back straight, as if it's up against a wall. Your bottom leg should be straight. Your top leg should be bent, with your foot flat on the floor in front of your bottom thigh.

2

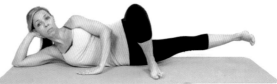

Inhale as you lengthen and lift your bottom leg off the mat a few inches.

3

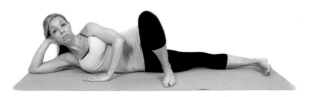

Exhale as you lower your bottom leg back to the mat. Repeat this exercise 10 times before repeating with your other leg.

CHALLENGE YOURSELF

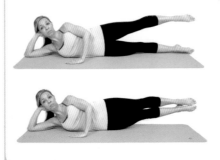

Lengthen your top leg long, in line with your hip, and hold still as you lift and lower your bottom leg to your top leg. This advanced variation works your inner thighs and challenges your core.

kneeling side kicks

The kneeling side kicks are a more-challenging variation of the leg sweep you learned in the side-lying exercises. When doing this exercise, the tendency is to cheat by letting your hip hinge to the back, which makes you lose part of the important core work. Therefore, make sure your body—your bottom knee, hips, spine, hand, and head—is in a straight line as viewed from the side.

{visualize} your torso staying stable as you kick your leg to the front and back.

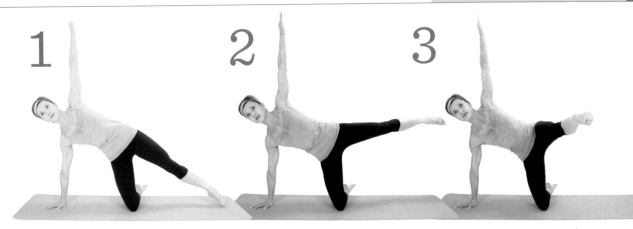

1 Kneel on one of your legs and bring your other leg straight out to the side with your toe on the mat. Place your hand on the floor and extend your other hand long to the ceiling.

2 Lift your extended leg off the floor at the same height as your hips with your foot pointed.

3 Inhale as you kick your leg to the front with a pointed foot, making sure your pelvis and torso are stable.

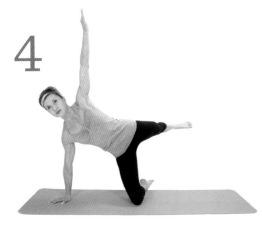

4 Exhale as you kick your leg to the back with a flexed foot. Repeat the sweeps 10 times before performing it with your other leg. Return to starting position.

MAKE IT EASIER

Hold the leg lift to strengthen your core.

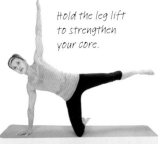

- Return to front and back sweeps to practice the leg sweeps in an easier torso position.

- Practice holding the leg lift in the center (10 to 30 seconds) until your core is strong enough to add the leg kicks.

KNEELING SIDE KICKS

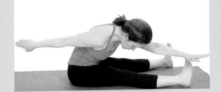

CHAPTER 6

Seated

You spend time every day in a sitting position. Therefore, this chapter contains exercises in a seated position to help strengthen and train your body for good alignment throughout the day. Keeping the Pilates scoop can be more challenging in a seated position, but remember, moving from your center is one of the Pilates principles. You may initially find it challenging to sit up straight and tall because of tightness in your hips or the back of your legs. If you do have trouble, bend your knees slightly or place a large block or book under your mat.

spine stretch

The focus of the spine stretch is the articulation of your spine. On the stretch forward, you start at the top of your spine with your head and neck. On the roll-up, you reverse the motion, getting your lower back in place first before rolling up through the rest of your spine. If your hamstrings are tight, you may feel a stretch along the back of the legs; feel free to bend your knees to focus only on your spine articulation.

BENEFITS

Develops spine articulation and control

Improves spine flexibility

Strengthens the muscles of the hips and core for sitting

{visualize} your arms reaching long on a track parallel to your legs.

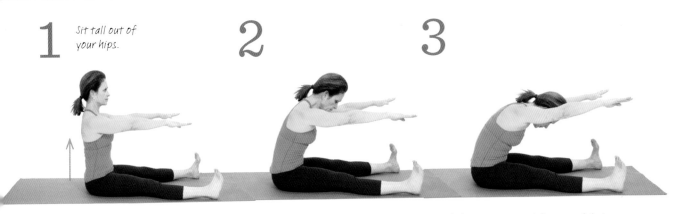

1 *Sit tall out of your hips.*

2

3

Sit tall with your legs in a small V-position and your arms stretched out in front of your shoulders.

Inhale as you prepare. Exhale as you start a C-curve through your spine by turning the top of your head forward.

Inhale as you stretch longer while in the C-curve.

4

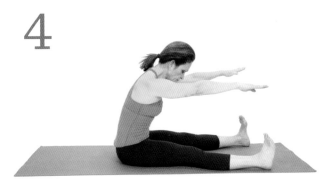

Exhale as you roll up, returning your lower back to sitting position and stacking each bone of your spine on top one at a time. Perform the exercise 10 times before returning to starting position.

MAKE IT EASIER

Sit with your knees bent.

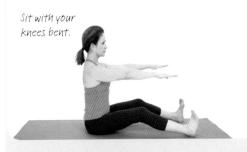

- Bend your knees to lessen the stretch on the back of your legs and to make it easier for you to sit tall.

- Sit on a block or in a chair to decrease the stretch on the back of your legs even more.

SPINE STRETCH

spine twist

The spine twist is beneficial for athletes in sports that require rotation, such as swinging a bat, racket, or club. Having your arms reaching out to your sides helps encourage a deeper rotation of your spine. Because your hips and legs are long on the mat, your lower body is stabilized to help isolate the rotation in your torso and spine.

BENEFITS

Develops oblique abdominal control

Improves spine flexibility and rotation

Strengthens the muscles of the hips and core for sitting

{visualize} your head as the pivot point for the motion.

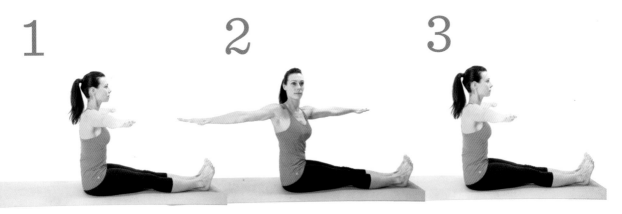

1

Sit tall with your legs together in front of your body and your feet flexed. Bring your arms out wide to your sides, palms down, with your hands a few inches in front of your shoulders at a slight angle to the front.

2

Slowly inhale to prepare as you grow your spine longer. Exhale as you rotate to one side, pivoting through the center of your head and spine as you rotate. Feel your waist engage and rotate, as if wringing out a towel.

3

Inhale as you rotate back to the center.

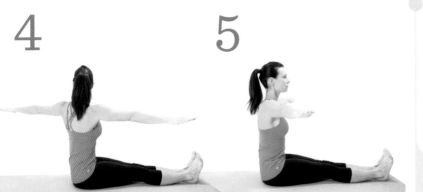

4

Exhale as you rotate to the other side.

5

Inhale as you rotate back to the center. Repeat the exercise 10 times, alternating the motion to each side, before returning to starting position.

MAKE IT EASIER

Sit with your legs in a V-position.

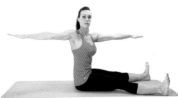

- Sit with your legs in a V-position for an easier leg position.

- Sit on a block or in a chair for less of a stretch to the back of your legs.

SPINE TWIST

saw

The saw is a combination of the spine twist and spine stretch exercises earlier in this chapter and concentrates on your spine and lower body. When doing this exercise, only reach as far as you are able, keeping both sides of your pelvis and hips down on the mat. You should also pay particular attention to the separation of your twist and forward reach.

BENEFITS

Improves spine and lower-body flexibility

Strengthens the muscles of the hips and core for sitting

Develops coordination

{visualize} your arm reaching forward and performing a small saw motion back and forth.

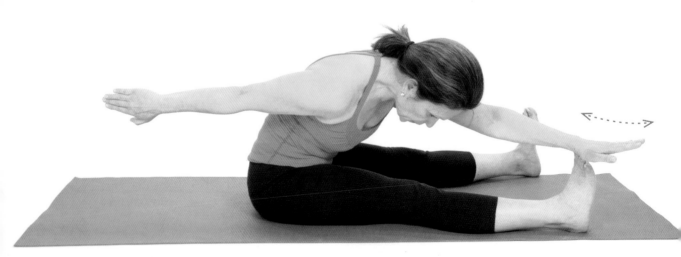

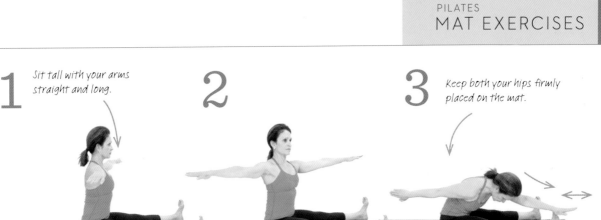

1 *Sit tall with your arms straight and long.*

2

3 *Keep both your hips firmly placed on the mat.*

Sit with your legs in a V-position, feet flexed. Bring your arms out horizontal to your sides, palms down.

Inhale as you rotate your body to the right side, pivoting through the top of your head.

Exhale as you reach your left hand to the outside of your right little toe, making sure your left hip doesn't roll off the mat. Look at your right knee while keeping your abdominals scooped. Perform 3 small reaches forward past your little toe, imagining your arm acting as a saw.

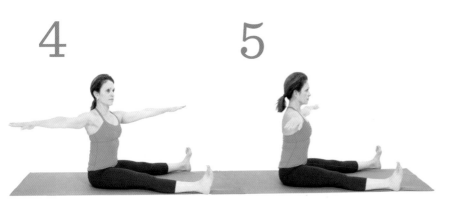

4

5

Inhale as you stack your spine and sit up in the rotated position.

Exhale as you rotate your spine back to the center and repeat to the other side. Repeat the exercise 10 times, alternating sides, before returning to starting position.

mermaid

The mermaid stretches your sides, ribcage, and shoulder. While performing this exercise, feel the space between your ribs opening and your waistline lengthening as you reach your arm overhead. In the side sit, your knees are close to your hips; if the mermaid side sit is uncomfortable for you, consider coming to the seated fourth described in the mermaid using a foam roller later in this book.

{visualize} your body being placed between two panes of glass as you stretch straight to the side.

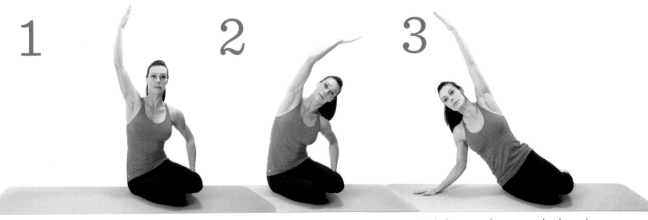

1

Sit with both your legs to the left side of your body, placing your heels close to your buttocks. Bring your right arm straight up to the ceiling.

2

Inhale as you stretch over your legs to your left, making sure you stretch straight to the side.

3

Exhale as you lower your body to the right side, placing your hand on the floor. Your spine should come to a straight position, with your left arm overhead.

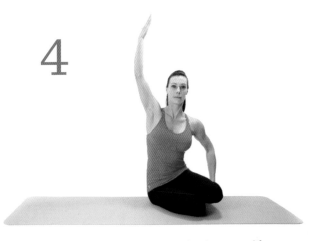

4

Inhale as you use your core and right arm to lift back to a sitting position while reaching your right arm up to the ceiling. Repeat the exercise 5 times before repeating on the other side.

● MAKE IT EASIER

Hold the stretch over your legs.

- Perform just the side stretch over your legs to do only the stretching portion of the mermaid.

- Come to a seated fourth position, with one leg bent at a right angle in front of your body and your other leg to the side, for an easier lower-body position.

MERMAID

can-can

The can-can is a nice stretch for the side of your hips and your spine. You also use your abdominals to initiate the movement of your legs. Although your arms are providing some support for your torso, be sure to use your core to keep your torso long and your lower back supported.

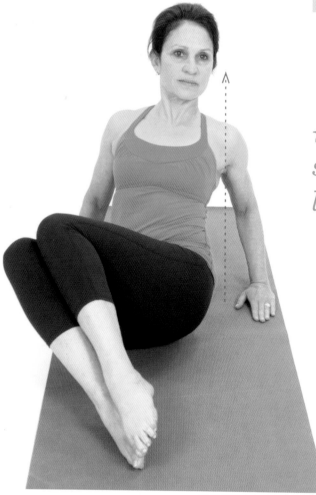

{visualize} your spine lengthening long.

1

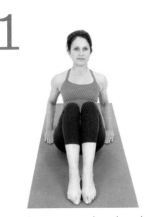

Sit with your arms placed on the mat behind you. Lean your torso slightly to the back, bend your legs to your chest, and point your toes. Have the tips of your toes gently rest on the floor.

2

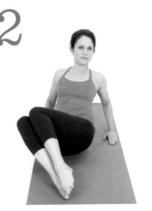

Inhale as you let your knees fall to one side, keeping your feet and knees pressed together.

3

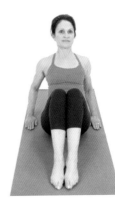

Exhale as you draw your legs back to the center using your core to move them.

4

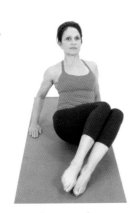

Inhale as you drop your knees to the other side. Exhale as you draw your legs back to the center. Repeat the exercise 10 times, alternating sides, before returning to starting position.

MAKE IT EASIER

Come down on your elbows.

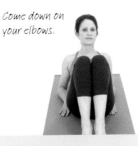

- Come down on your elbows for a lower torso position and more support.
- Keep your knee drop to the side small for less of a stretch and less work for your abdominals.

modified hip circles

Hip circles are one of the most-challenging Pilates mat exercises. This modified version of hip circles requires lower-body and upper-body flexibility and core control. If you were doing full hip circles, your legs would stay straight for the entire motion and your feet would make a circle; for this exercise, your legs are bent before straightening to draw an arch from one side to the other. If the backs of your legs are tight, keep your knees lightly bent.

BENEFITS

Strengthens the abdominals

Improves upper-body flexibility

Challenges balance

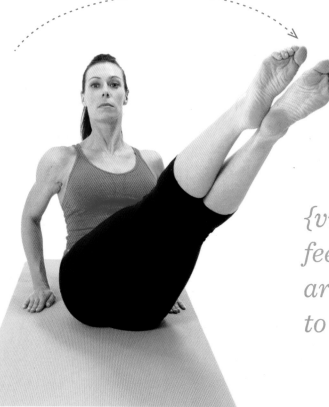

{visualize} your feet drawing an arch from one side to the other.

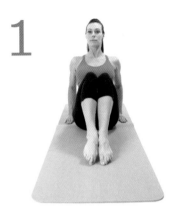

1

Sit with your arms placed on the mat behind you. Lean your torso slightly to the back, bend your legs to your chest, and point your toes. Have the tips of your toes gently rest on the floor.

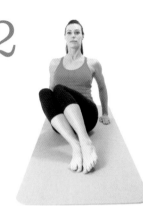

2

Inhale as you let your knees fall to one side.

3

Exhale as you extend your legs to the side and press your feet together.

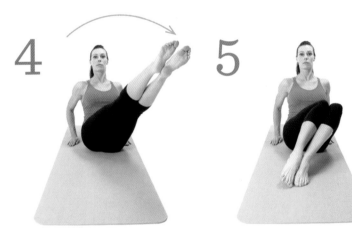

4

Inhale as you draw an arch with your legs to the ceiling and over to the other side.

5

Exhale as you bend your knees and place your feet on the floor. Repeat the exercise 5 times one direction before reversing directions. Return to starting position.

CHALLENGE YOURSELF

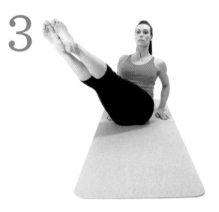

Keep your legs straight throughout the entire circle.

Hold your legs straight the entire time, letting your feet draw a circle for the full, unmodified hip circle.

MODIFIED HIP CIRCLES

seated fourth glute work

As the name says, this exercise is great for working your glutes. The positioning during the seated fourth glute work is particularly important, as it isolates your glute muscles. To do it properly, you should have the knee of your working leg in line with your hip. If your knee is in front of your hip, you are likely using your hip flexors instead of your glutes to lift your leg.

BENEFITS

Strengthens the glutes

Challenges balance

Develops coordination

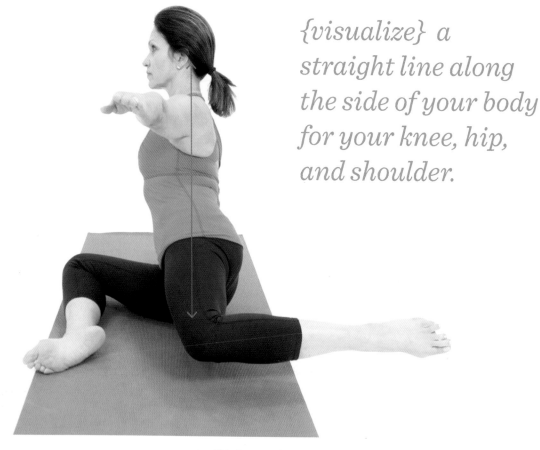

{visualize} a straight line along the side of your body for your knee, hip, and shoulder.

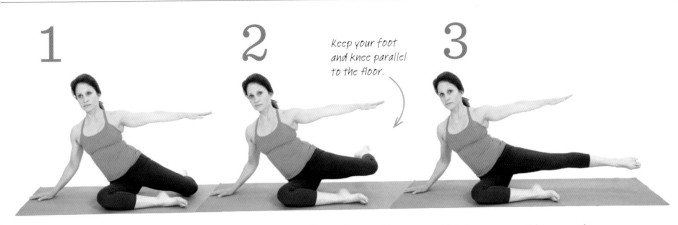

Keep your foot and knee parallel to the floor.

1 Sit with one leg bent at a 90-degree angle in front of your body. Bend your other leg at a 90-degree angle straight out to your side, with your knee in line with your hip. Sit up tall with your hand resting on the floor.

2 Inhale as you lift your foot and knee off the mat.

3 Exhale as you straighten your knee, keeping your thigh lifted.

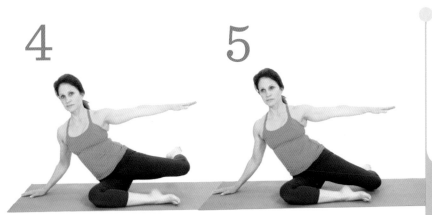

4 Inhale as you bend your knee, still keeping your thigh lifted.

5 Exhale as you lower your thigh back to the mat. Repeat the exercise 10 times before repeating it with your other leg.

CHALLENGE YOURSELF

Hold your arms out to your sides.

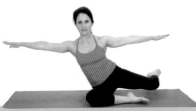

- Attempt the exercise with both arms extended to your sides for more of a challenge to your balance.

- Hold a bent leg in a lifted position and do small, pulsing reaches to the ceiling or to the back for more-isolated glute work.

SEATED FOURTH GLUTE WORK

115

circles in the sand

Circles in the sand provides a good stretch to your back and hips. Your fingertips drag along the floor, as if drawing a "circle in the sand." As you perform this exercise, keep your abdominals scooped and both your hips firmly planted on the mat.

BENEFITS

Stretches the back and hips
Develops abdominal scoop
Improves spine flexibility

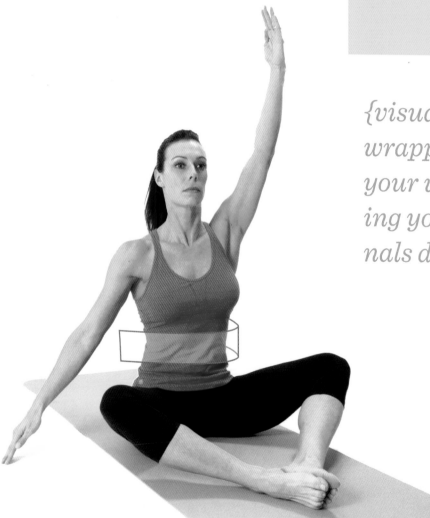

{visualize} a band wrapped around your waist, keeping your abdominals drawn in.

1

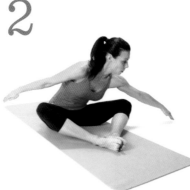

The bottom of your feet should be pressing together.

Sit on the mat with your knees bent at a 90-degree angle in a butterfly position. Have your inner thighs slightly engaged and your arms at your sides with your fingertips near the floor.

2

Inhale as you reach one arm to the back and begin drawing a circle with your fingertips near the floor.

3

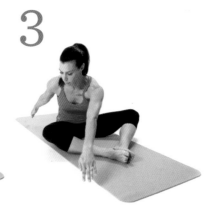

On a long exhale, continue drawing the circle near the floor with your fingertips to the front of your feet and over to the other side.

4

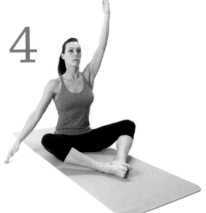

One you have drawn a circle as far as you can, inhale as you lift your arm overhead.

5

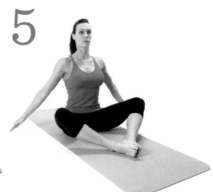

Exhale as you lower your arm back to the floor. Repeat the circle with your other arm. Repeat the exercise 10 times, alternating sides.

CIRCLES IN THE SAND

CHAPTER 7

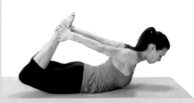

On Your Stomach

This chapter contains exercises done on your stomach, which help strengthen the back of your body. The traditional Pilates work includes advanced exercises like the swan dive and the rocker, where you maintain your body in an arced position while rolling on the front of your torso; here, I will walk you through just the swan and rocker position and use them as exercises in and of themselves.

During all of these exercises, be careful to support your spine by keeping your Pilates scoop. Keeping your navel to your spine will allow you to avoid overextending your back by keeping your lower back in the same arc you would have in a standing posture. As you extend your back, think of coming to a smooth arc, instead of an arch, to avoid extending too far.

single-leg kick

The single-leg kick strengthens the back of your legs and glutes while the front of your leg is stretched. During the exercise, your upper body should be positioned with your weight on your elbows and forearms, with your shoulders down and away from your ears. As you are up on your elbows, make sure you support your lower back but still keep your abdominals engaged by drawing your navel up and away from the floor.

{visualize} a string pulling your heel toward your buttocks as you bend your knee.

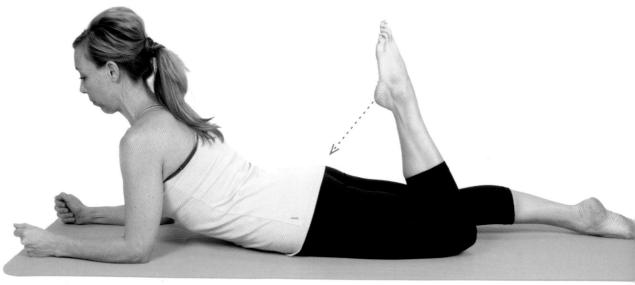

1 *Keep your neck in line with the rest of your spine.*

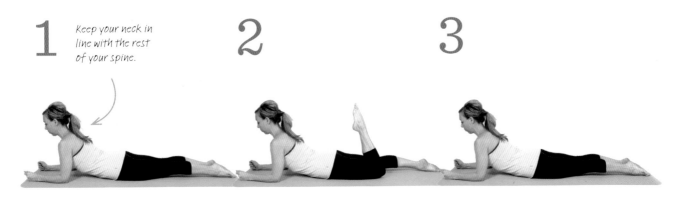

Lie on your stomach propped on your elbows. Press your shoulders down and away from your ears.

2

Inhale as you beat your left heel toward your buttocks twice.

3

Exhale as you lower your leg down to the mat.

4

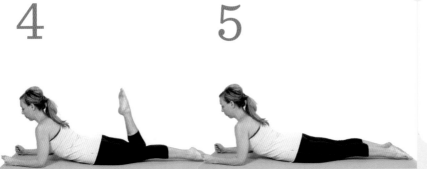

Inhale as you beat your right heel toward your buttocks twice.

5

Exhale as you lower your leg down to the mat. Repeat the exercise 10 times, alternating sides.

MAKE IT EASIER

Rest your head on your hands.

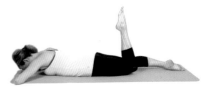

- Lower your torso down to the mat, resting your head on your hands with your elbows bent to the sides. This gives you an easier position for your torso and upper body.

- Omit the two heel beats toward the buttocks and practice just the knee bend with control for a simplified version of the exercise.

SINGLE-LEG KICK

121

double-leg kick

During the double-leg kick, both your legs work as a unit as your heels beat toward your buttocks and your legs extend, working your glutes and the back of your legs. You also vary which way your head is turned and placed on the mat for an alternating neck stretch. Note that when your legs extend and lengthen, you turn your head through the center to the other side as your arms extend behind you.

BENEFITS

Strengthens the glutes and back of the legs

Strengthens the upper back

Stretches the shoulders, neck, and front of the thighs

{visualize} your upper back arcing as your arms reach to the back.

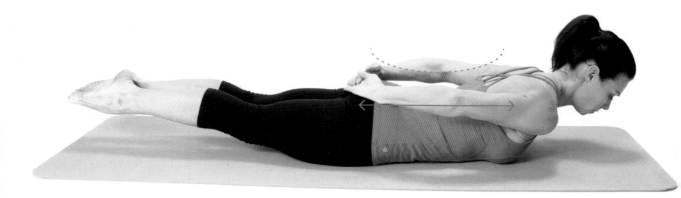

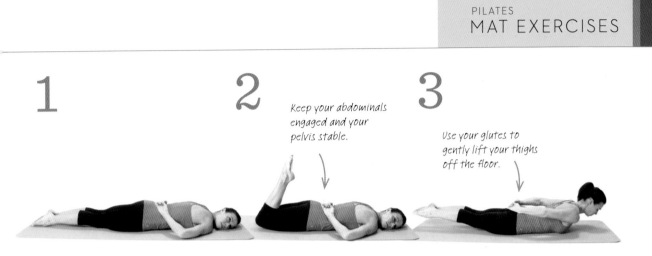

1

Lie on the mat with your head turned to one side. Put your hands together on the small of your back and have your legs lengthened long on the mat behind you.

2

Keep your abdominals engaged and your pelvis stable.

Inhale as you beat your heels toward your buttocks twice.

3

Use your glutes to gently lift your thighs off the floor.

Exhale as you extend your legs and lift your thighs off the floor. At the same time, turn your head to the center, reach your arms toward your feet, and lift your upper torso off the mat.

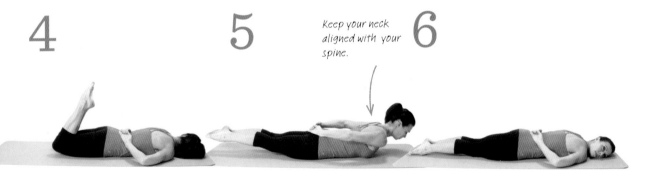

4

Turn your head to the other side and lower your legs and torso to the mat. Inhale as you beat your heels toward your buttocks twice.

5

Keep your neck aligned with your spine.

Exhale as you extend your legs and lift your thighs off the floor. At the same time, turn your head to the center, reach your arms toward your feet, and lift your upper torso off the mat.

6

Turn your head to the other side and lower your legs and torso to the mat. Repeat the exercise 10 times before finishing in the starting position.

DOUBLE-LEG KICK

swimming

Swimming strengthens the muscles of your core and back as you move both of your arms and legs while holding your torso stable. As you perform this exercise, move your arms and legs briskly as you breathe deeply with 5 counts of inhalation and 5 counts of exhalation. This brisk movement helps activate your cardiovascular system.

{visualize} your shoulder blades sliding down into your back pockets.

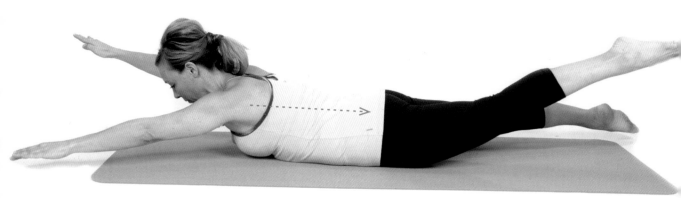

1

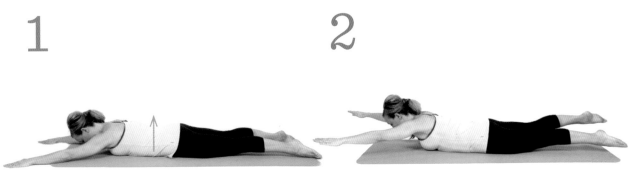

Lie on your stomach with your arms over your head and your legs on the mat behind you. Inhale as you pull your navel toward your spine.

2

Exhale as you lift both your arms and legs off the mat. Arc your upper back slightly while continuing to look at the floor. Feel a long line from the top of your head to the tips of your toes.

3

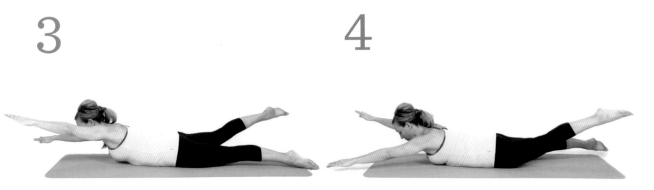

Begin beating your arms and legs briskly, as if paddling in water. Start the beats by raising your left arm and right leg.

4

Lower your left arm and right leg as your opposite limbs lift. Do 5 paddles on an inhale and 5 paddles on the exhale. Repeat for 5 sets of breaths. Return to starting position by lowering your upper body, arms, and legs back to the mat.

swan

The swan stretches the front of your body and strengthens your back. To avoid overextending when doing this exercise, use your abdominals to stabilize your lower back. Focus the arcing of your back to the middle of your back instead of your lower back or neck, as these two areas naturally have an extension curve at rest. When you extend high off the mat, the front of your pelvis should be lifted off the mat.

BENEFITS

Strengthens the back

Improves spine extension

Stretches the muscles on the front of the body

{visualize} your breastbone lifting to the ceiling.

1

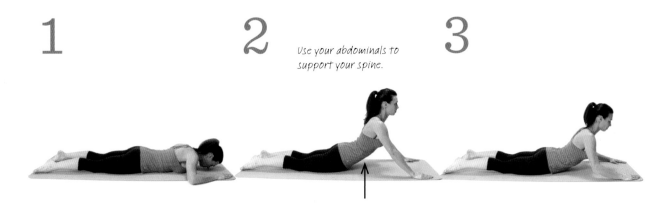

Lie on your stomach with your hands to the sides of your body and your elbows bent.

2

Use your abdominals to support your spine.

Inhale as you draw your shoulder blades into your back pockets. Begin lifting your head and chest, as if you're a turtle sticking its head out of its shell. Continue lifting by pressing your hands into the mat until you're in an extended position.

3

Exhale as you bend your arms and begin lowering back to the mat.

4

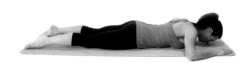

Continue exhaling as you lower all the way down to the mat. Repeat 5 times to finish in starting position.

CHALLENGE YOURSELF

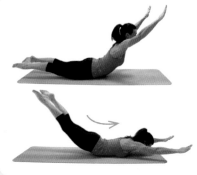

Perform the swan dive, in which your body holds a swan position while you rock from your chest to your thighs, inhaling as you rock forward and exhaling as you rock back. The swan dive is an advanced exercise that challenges your entire body.

SWAN

swan with neck rolls

During the swan with neck rolls, you hold a swan position as you move your neck while your shoulders, torso, and hips remain stable. This provides a good stretch for your neck and the front of your body. When performing this exercise, be careful to only move in a range that is comfortable for you as you do it both clockwise and counterclockwise.

BENEFITS

Strengthens the back

Stretches the muscles in the front of the body and neck

Improves spine extension

{visualize} your nose drawing a semicircle.

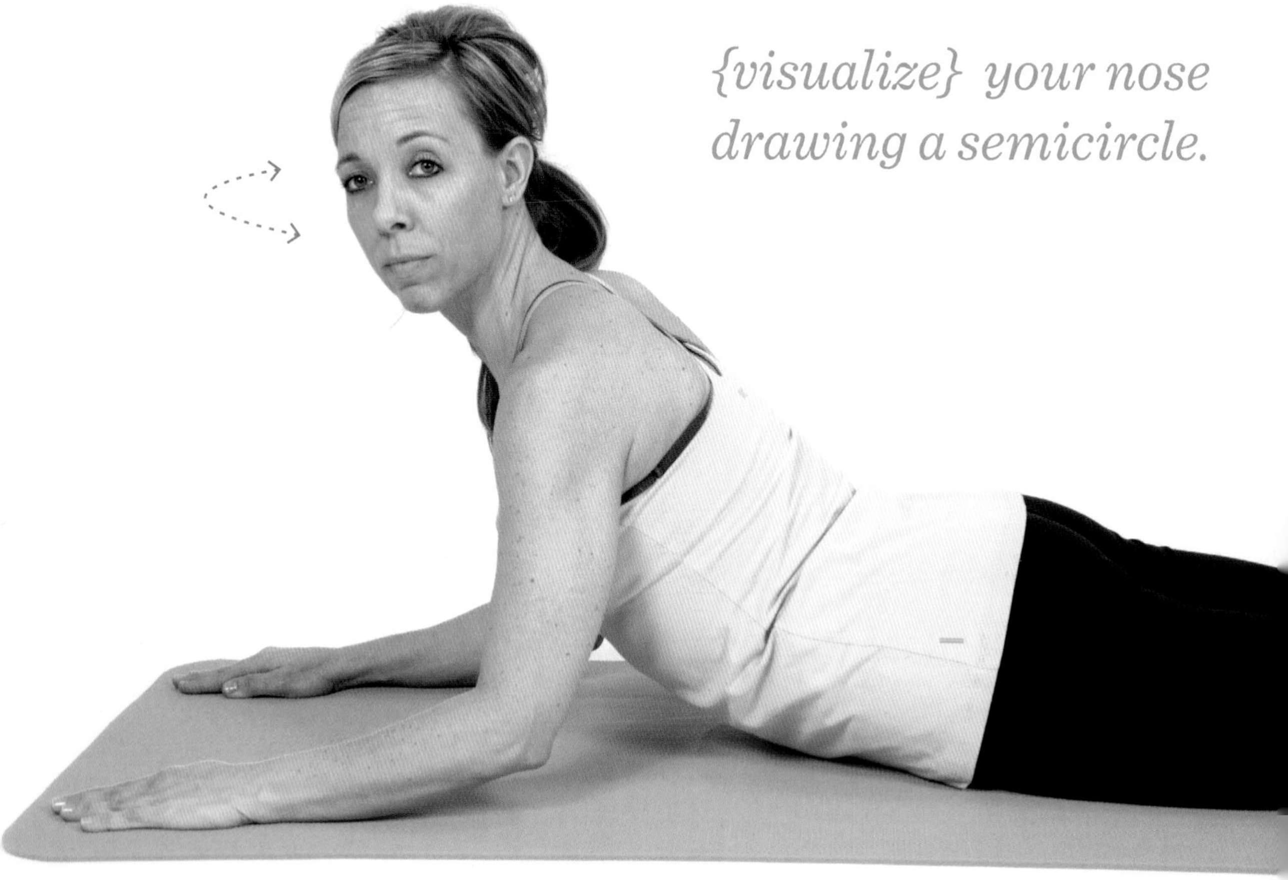

1

2

Keep your gluteal muscles and the back of your legs engaged.

3

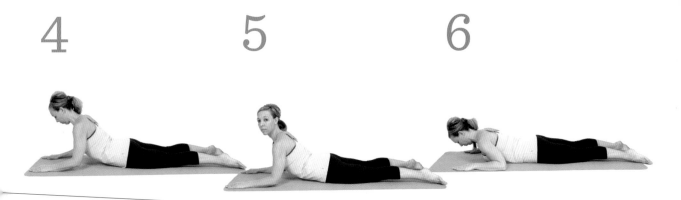

Lie on your stomach with your hands to the sides of your body and your elbows bent. Inhale as you slide your shoulder blades down your back and engage your core.

Exhale as you lift your head and chest. Continue lifting by pressing your hands into the mat until you are in an extended position.

Holding an extended position, inhale as you turn your head to one side.

4

5

6

Exhale as you draw your chin to your chest while turning your head to the other side.

Inhale as you turn your head to the other side. Exhale as you turn your head back to the center. Repeat the circle 3 times.

After 3 circles, exhale as you lower your torso back to the mat. Repeat the exercise 5 times in the other direction and return to starting position.

rocker position

The rocker is an advanced exercise where your body rocks from your chest to your thighs while holding an extended position. In this version, I teach you how to get into the rocker position and hold it. The rocker position is a great stretch for the front of your body, including your quadriceps, abdominals, and shoulders.

BENEFITS

Stretches the front of the torso and thighs

Stretches the shoulders and chest

Strengthens the back

{visualize} your body balancing on your pelvis as you hold the rocker position.

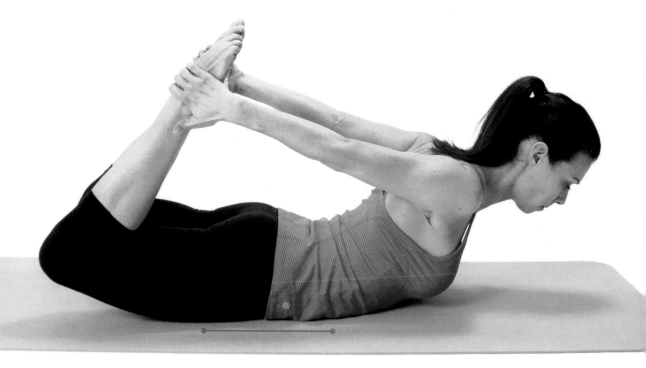

CHAPTER 7 • ON YOUR STOMACH

1

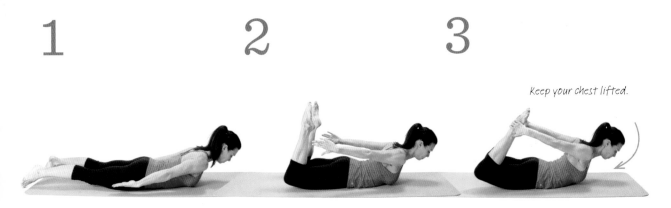

Lie on your stomach. Inhale as you arc your upper back, lifting your head and neck off the mat.

2

Exhale as you extend your arms behind you and bend your knees. Grab onto your ankles, if able, to hold the rocker position.

3

Keep your chest lifted.

Breathe for 5 inhales and 5 exhales as you feel the front of your thighs, abdominals, and front of your shoulders stretch.

4

5

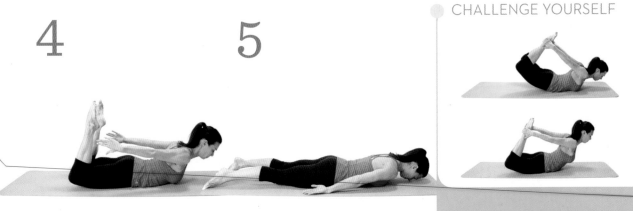

Inhale as you let go of your ankles.

Exhale as you straighten your knees and lower your torso and legs back down to the mat.

CHALLENGE YOURSELF

Do the full rocker exercise by rocking forward to your chest on an inhalation and rocking back onto your thighs on an exhalation.

ROCKER POSITION

heel beats

The heel beats are quick, small movements that work the back of your legs and glutes. I typically have my clients start with 5 beats on inhalations and 5 beats on exhalations, as shown here. During this exercise, to protect your back, make sure your core stays engaged as you keep both your legs lengthened off the mat.

BENEFITS

Strengthens the glutes and inner thighs

Challenges the core

Develops coordination

{visualize} your thighs and glutes squeezing together.

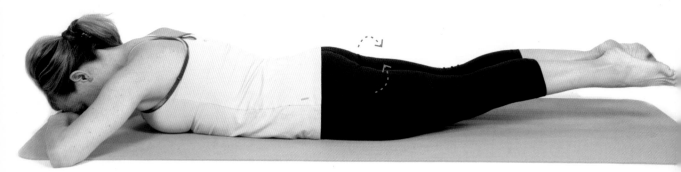

1

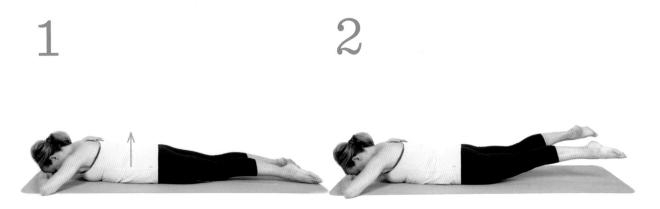

Lie on your stomach with your arms bent and your palms down on the mat. Rest your head on your hands. Inhale as you engage your core, drawing your navel to your spine.

2

Exhale as you lift your legs slightly off the mat, keeping your knees straight and feet pointed.

3

Use your inner thighs and glutes to beat your heels in a small, quick movement.

Beat your heels together for 5 inhalations and 5 exhalations. Repeat for 5 sets of breaths.

4

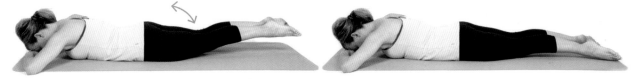

Inhale and exhale as you lower your legs back to the mat to return to starting position.

CHAPTER 8

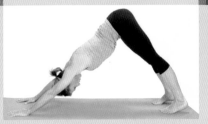

Planks and All Fours

Planks are some of the most intense Pilates exercises. In this chapter, aside from the all-fours exercise the cat, you'll find that plank exercises are a great challenge for your entire body. If you feel the full-front and side plank positions are too difficult at first, practice planks in a modified position on your knees or simply do part of the exercise. Take your time learning the exercises in this chapter.

all fours to plank

You'll use the all fours to plank—which is a great strengthener for your core, abdominals, and upper body—as a transition into and out of your front-plank positions. Here, you use the motion as an exercise to practice. As you do this, your shoulders and hips should stay square and stable—avoid letting your hips and torso rotate or rock from side to side as you move your legs.

BENEFITS

Strengthens the core and abdominals

Strengthens the upper body

Develops core stabilization

{visualize} your hips and shoulders staying stable like a board.

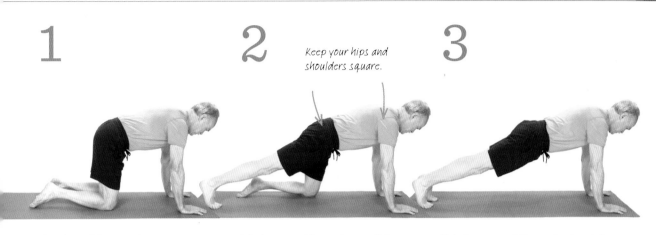

1

Kneel on all fours with your spine straight.

2

Keep your hips and shoulders square.

Inhale as you lift one knee off the floor and extend the ball of your foot on the floor behind you. This position begins your plank position.

3

Exhale as you shift your bodyweight to your arms and the ball of your foot behind you to bring your other leg to a plank position.

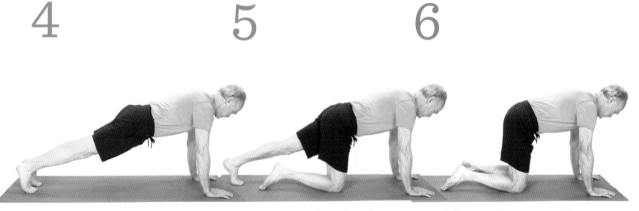

4

Hold the plank position for one slow breath, feeling a long line from your feet to your head.

5

Inhale as you bend one knee back to the floor to begin returning to the all-fours position.

6

Exhale as you bring your other knee back to the floor to return to starting position. Repeat the exercise 5 times.

cat

The cat is a stretch for your back that focuses on spine artic-ulation. When you round your spine, start with a pelvic curl, beginning the round at the bottom of your spine. To length-en, start at the bottom of your spine once again by turning your tailbone to the back of the room. Once in a lengthened position, the curves in your spine should be the same as if you're in a standing position.

BENEFITS

Stretches the back

Develops spine articulation

Improves abdominal control

{visualize} a band wrapped around your waist, pulling your spine up to the ceiling as you round.

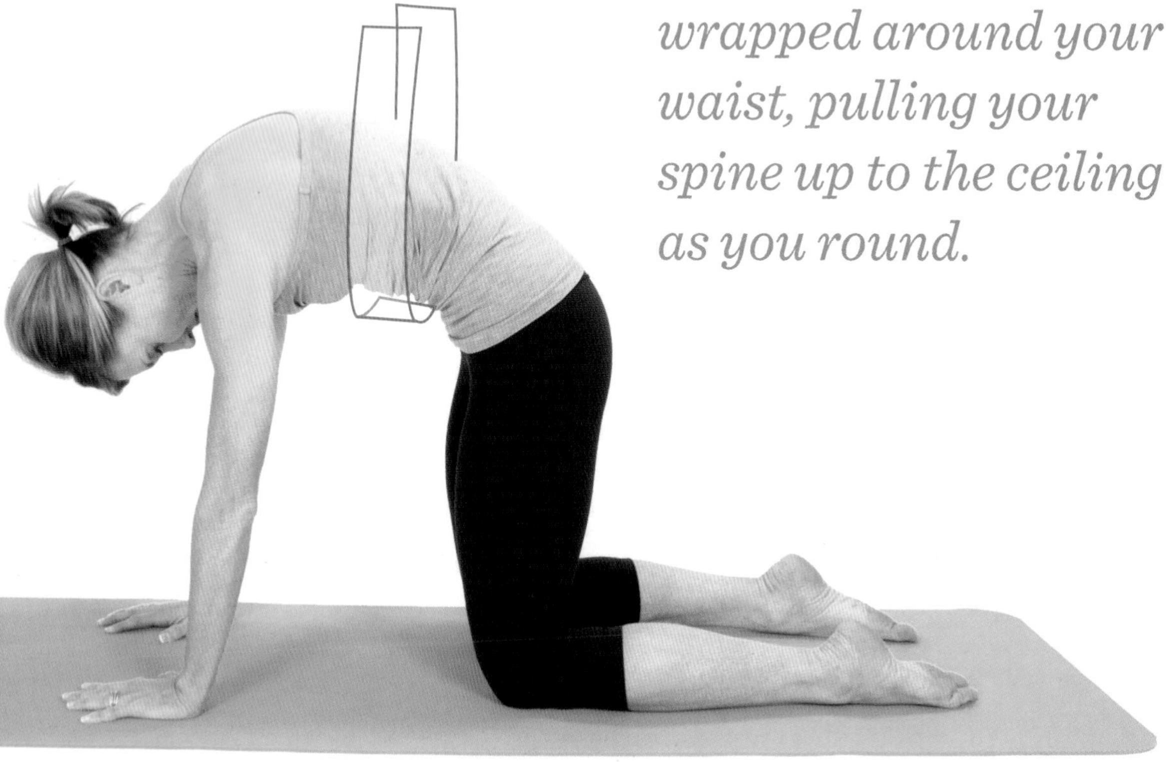

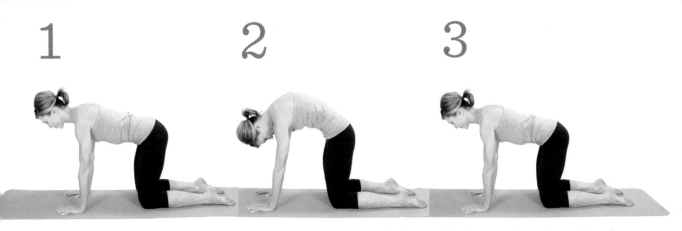

1

Position yourself on all fours with your knees directly under your hips and your hands under your shoulders. Have your spine long, as if you're in a standing position.

2

Inhale as you start a pelvic curl and round your spine. Continue rounding your spine in your lower back, then your midback, and finally your neck and head.

3

Exhale as you release the pelvic curl, lengthening your tailbone behind you. Let your spine grow long from your tailbone to your head and return to starting position. Repeat the exercise 5 times.

MAKE IT EASIER

Draw your navel toward your spine.

CHALLENGE YOURSELF

Use your core muscles to hover your knees off the mat.

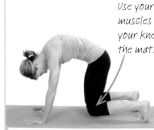

- Practice articulating your spine while sitting in a chair to practice the cat stretch without the upper-body challenge of being on your knees.
- While on all fours, hold a long, straight spine and try drawing your navel to your spine to practice a part of the exercise and your Pilates scoop.

Extend your toes on the mat so the ball of your foot is on the floor. As you round, scoop so deeply that your knees lift off the floor. Hold your knees in this position with your core engaged for 30 seconds to strengthen your core and arms.

CAT

leg pull front

During the leg pull front, you hold a plank facing the floor and lift your legs off the floor, keeping your pelvis in a line between your shoulders and feet. Holding stable while lifting your legs provides a challenge that strengthens your core and upper body. You should feel your hands pressing into the floor to keep your shoulder blades positioned well on your back.

{visualize} your pelvis staying positioned between your shoulders and feet.

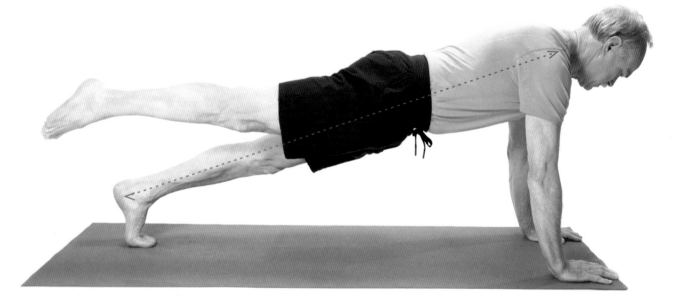

1

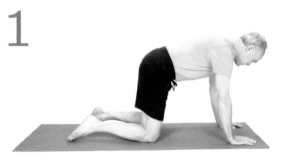

Begin on all fours. Use the all fours to plank exercise in this chapter to get into a plank position.

2

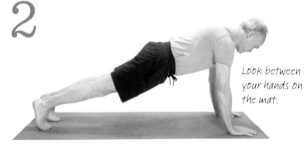

Look between your hands on the mat.

Hold a stable plank position with your shoulders broad and your hips in line with your shoulders and feet.

3

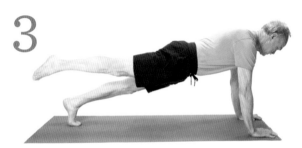

Inhale as you lift one leg off the floor, pointing your foot.

4

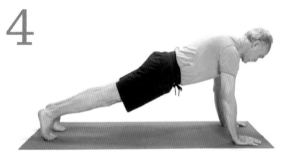

Exhale as you lower your leg back to the floor.

5

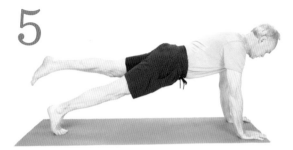

Inhale as you lift your other leg off the floor, pointing your foot.

6

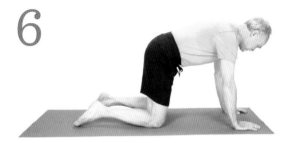

Exhale as you lower your leg back to the floor. Repeat the leg lifts 10 times, alternating legs, and return back to starting position using the all fours to plank exercise.

push-up

The push-up—which strengthens your core, abdominals, and upper body—starts and ends in a standing position. This exercise combines the standing rolldown exercise, a V-stretch position, a front plank, and a push-up into one continuous motion. As you transition from the rolldown to the plank, use your core to keep your torso centered on the mat.

{visualize} your shoulder blades remaining stable on your back during the push-up.

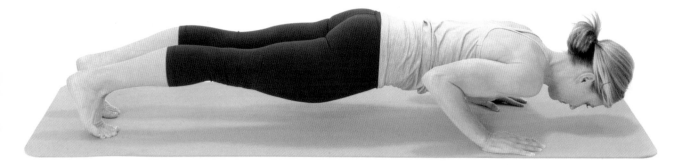

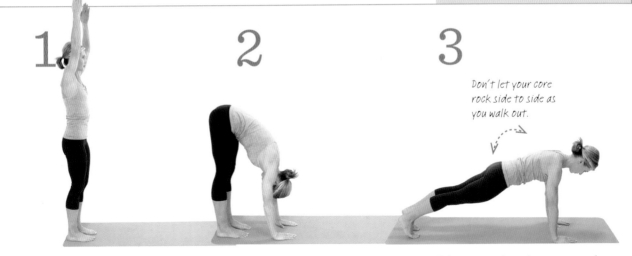

1 Stand at the end of the mat. Inhale as you bring your arms overhead.

2 Exhale as you roll down your spine, articulating one bone at a time. Keep your abdominals scooped as your spine comes to a C-shape. Place your hands on the floor.

3 *Don't let your core rock side to side as you walk out.*

Take as many breaths as you need as you walk out to a plank position.

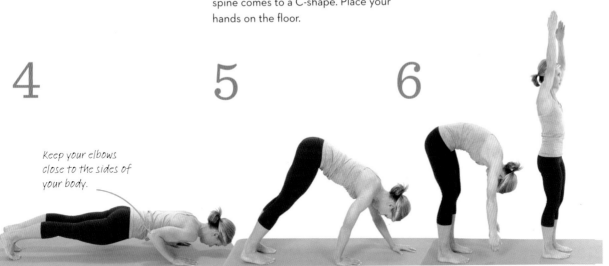

4 *Keep your elbows close to the sides of your body.*

Once in a plank, inhale as you bend your elbows, doing a push-up motion. Exhale as you push your arms into a plank position.

5 Walk your hands back toward your feet as your hips lift up.

6 Roll back to a standing position, getting your pelvis in place first and then growing tall through the rest of your spine. Repeat the exercise 5 times and finish in a standing position.

leg pullback

The leg pullback uses a similar sequence to the leg pull front, only now you position yourself with your body facing the ceiling. You use upper-body strength to keep your shoulder blades down and away from your ears, and you use your gluteal and core strength to keep your hips lifted. During this exercise, keep the back of your legs engaged, being careful to avoid letting your knees hyperextend on the leg lifts.

{visualize} a straight line for your feet, hips, and shoulders.

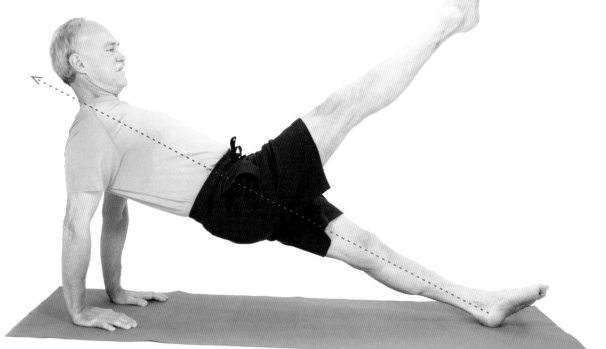

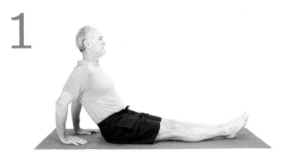

1

Sit with your legs straight and together on the mat. Place your hands behind you flat on the floor with your fingers facing your body.

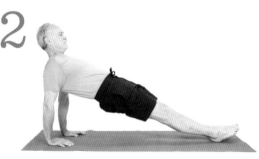

2

Inhale as you slide your shoulder blades down your back and shift your weight onto your hands. Exhale as you lift your hips off the mat, coming to a straight reverse-plank position.

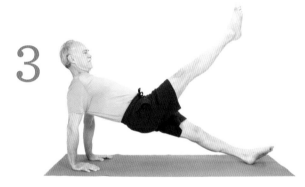

3

Inhale as you lift one leg to the ceiling, only lifting as far as you are able to while keeping your core stable.

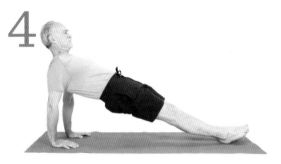

4

Exhale as you lower your leg back to the floor.

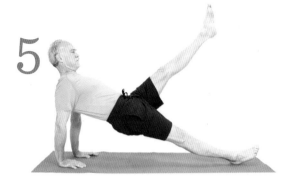

5

Inhale as you lift your other leg to the ceiling.

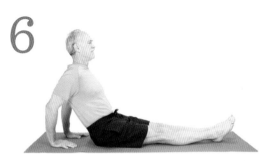

6

Exhale as you lower your leg back to the floor. Repeat the exercise 10 times, alternating sides. Lower your hips back to the mat with one breath cycle to return to starting position.

side bend

The side bend strengthens and stretches the side of your body. Your top arm moves the same direction as your hips—reaching overhead on the hip lift and coming down by your side on the hip drop. As you perform this, focus on keeping your bottom shoulder in good alignment and down and away from your ear during both your hip lift and drop.

{visualize} your hips lifting to the ceiling on the side bend when you reach overhead.

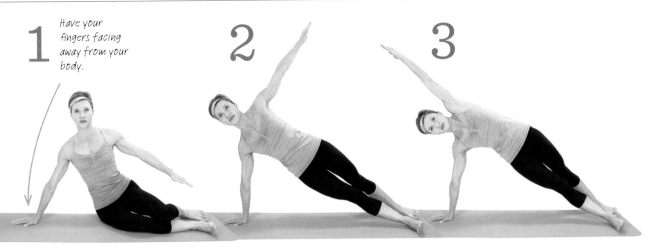

1 *Have your fingers facing away from your body.*

Sit with your legs slightly bent. Move your top leg to the back. Align your feet, hips, shoulder, and hand in a straight line on the mat. Inhale to prepare.

2

To get in position for the side lifts, exhale as you lift your hips off the mat, supporting your body with your feet and your bottom arm. Take your nonsupporting arm straight up to the ceiling.

3

Inhale as you press your hips to the ceiling while your top arm turns to reach overhead. You should feel the long stretch and side bend through your body.

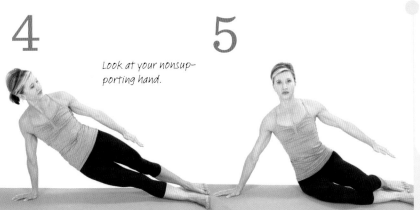

4 *Look at your nonsupporting hand.*

Exhale as you lower your hips toward the mat, bringing your nonsupporting arm to the side of your torso. Repeat the side lifts 5 times.

5

Bend your knees and lower your hips back down to the mat. Repeat the exercise on the other side.

MAKE IT EASIER

Come to a side plank on your knee.

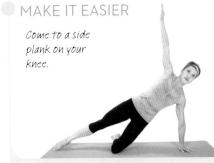

- Hold a side plank on your knee, with your top leg lengthened long to the side, for an easier upper-body and core position.
- Practice holding a full side plank until strong enough to do the hip lifts and drops.

SIDE BEND

twist

During the twist, you move from a side-plank position and rotate your hips to the ceiling as you dive your hand down to the mat. Similar to the side bend, this works your core, upper body, and side. During this challenging core exercise, keep the shoulder of your supporting arm positioned well to avoid placing stress on it.

{visualize} your hips lifting to the ceiling as you twist.

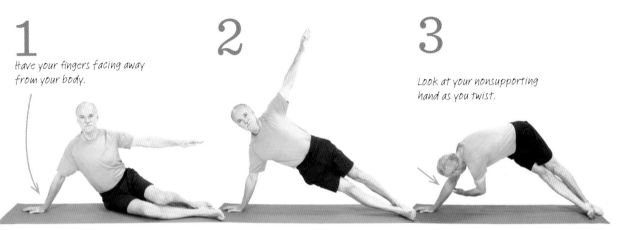

1

Have your fingers facing away from your body.

Sit with your legs slightly bent. Move your top leg to the back. Align your feet, hips, shoulder, and hand in a straight line on the mat. Inhale to prepare.

2

To get in position for the torso twist, exhale as you lift your hips off the mat, supporting your body with your feet and your bottom arm. Take your nonsupporting arm straight up to the ceiling.

3

Look at your nonsupporting hand as you twist.

Inhale as you lift your hips to the ceiling and rotate to bring your nonsupporting hand just behind your supporting hand.

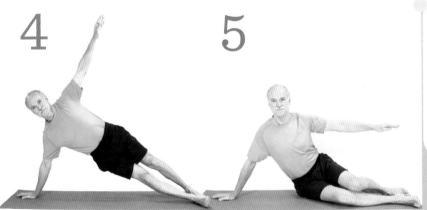

4

Exhale as you lower your hips toward the mat and rotate back to face the front. Repeat the torso twist 5 times.

5

Bend your knees and lower your hips back down to the mat. Repeat the exercise on the other side.

CHALLENGE YOURSELF

Look at your top hand.

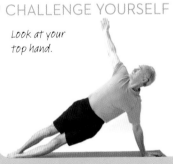

- Hold a side plank and keep your pelvis stable as you rotate for more focus on the rotation of your upper body and spine during the twist.

- Look up at your hand with each twist for more of a challenge to your balance.

plank to v-stretch

The plank to V-stretch both strengthens your core and stretches your body. Use your lower core to initiate a hinge at your hip as you lift your hips to the ceiling. Your body will then form an upside-down V-position—hence the name, V-stretch. Throughout the exercise, keep your spine as straight as you are able to in order to focus the stretch on your hips and legs.

BENEFITS

Strengthens the core and abdominals

Strengthens the upper body

Stretches the back of the legs and hips

Stretches the shoulders

{visualize} your body forming an upside-down V.

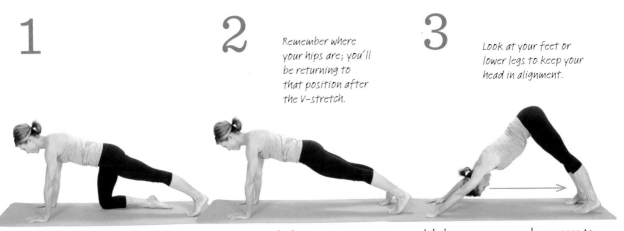

1

Begin on all fours. Use the all fours to plank exercise in this chapter to get into a plank position.

2

Remember where your hips are; you'll be returning to that position after the V-stretch.

Once in a plank, engage your core.

3

Look at your feet or lower legs to keep your head in alignment.

Inhale as you use your lower core to lift your hips to the ceiling. Let your heels reach down toward the floor and have your ears come between your arms.

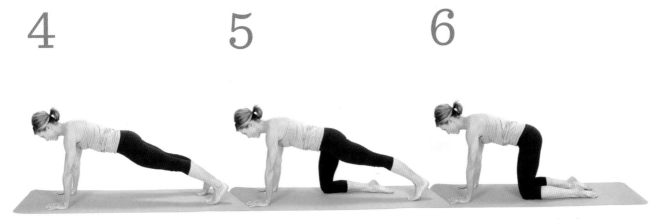

4

Exhale as you keep your spine straight and return to a plank position; be careful only to lower your hips to a position where they are in line with your shoulders and feet. Repeat this movement 10 times.

5

Come out of the plank position using the all fours to plank exercise. Inhale as you bend one knee back to the all-fours position.

6

Exhale as you bend your other leg back to the all-fours position.

CHAPTER 9

Standing

Like sitting, standing is something you do many times a day. This chapter is your opportunity to practice in a standing position! Training and strengthening your body in other positions is beneficial for your body, but these movement patterns of standing need to be integrated into your daily posture. To do the work correctly, awareness of the alignment and position of your body relative to gravity is important. While this chapter contains only a few exercises, you'll find equipment exercises in Part 3 that can also be done in a standing position.

standing rolldown

The standing rolldown is a similar motion to the roll-up, except you are now standing instead of lying on the mat. The rolldown starts at the top with your upper body and ends with the turn of your pelvis—a true workout for your spine. To perform this, it's important to have your pelvis in position on the roll back up so your spine has something to stack on top of.

{visualize} your spine stacking one bone at a time, as if your back is up against a wall.

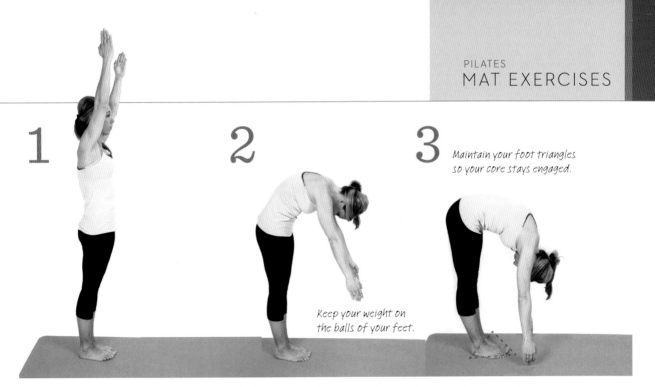

1

2

3 *Maintain your foot triangles so your core stays engaged.*

Keep your weight on the balls of your feet.

Stand with your feet together and your arms relaxed at your sides. Inhale as you bring your arms overhead.

Exhale as you reach your arms long and roll your head, neck, and shoulders down toward the mat, making sure your weight doesn't shift to your heels.

Take as many breaths as you need as you roll down toward the mat. Inhale as you hold at the bottom of the roll.

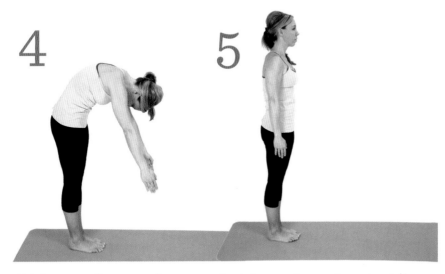

4

5

Exhale as you roll up to standing alignment, turning at your pelvis while scooping your lower abdominals.

Stack the rest of your spine on top, taking as many breaths as you need to complete the roll-up. Repeat the exercise 5 times before returning to a standing position.

shoulder shrugs

The muscles of your neck and shoulders are a common place to hold muscle tension. Shoulder shrugs use the motion of your shoulders and matching breathing patterns to gently contract and relax the muscles in those places. The rolling motion of your shoulders to the back encourages you to open your chest, thus correcting tight forward-rounded shoulders.

BENEFITS

Relaxes the shoulders and neck

Improves posture

Connects breath to movement

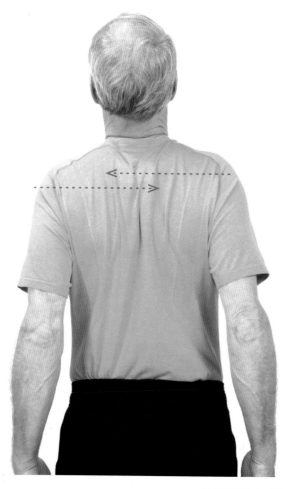

{visualize} your shoulder blades sliding together as you gently pull your shoulders back.

CHAPTER 9 • STANDING

1

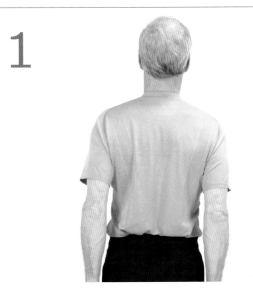

Get in a standing position with your arms resting at your sides.

2

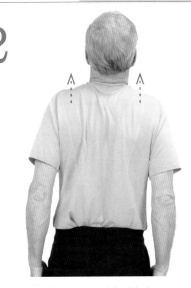

Inhale as you lift your shoulder blades up toward your ears.

3

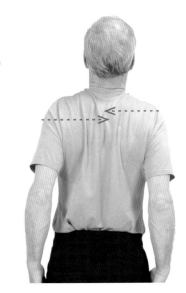

Start a long exhale as you squeeze your shoulder blades gently toward your spine.

4

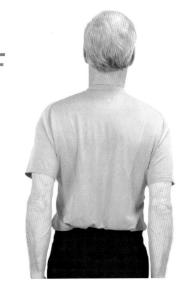

Continue to exhale as you let your shoulders lower down and away from your ears. Finish the exhale by allowing your shoulders to return to resting alignment. Repeat 5 times before returning to starting position.

SHOULDER SHRUGS

foot rolls and toe lifts

The feet are not only important for standing and walking, but also contain about 25 percent of the bones in your body. Foot rolls and toe lifts work on your foot triangles and your awareness of your foot alignment. As you perform these exercises, notice how the small changes in your feet can have a large impact on the alignment of the rest of your body.

BENEFITS

Improves alignment of the feet

Gently challenges balance

Strengthens the muscles of the lower leg

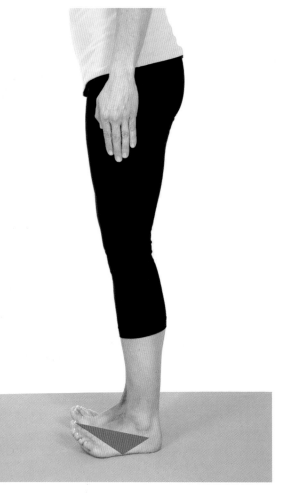

{visualize} triangles on the bottom of your feet during foot rolls and toe lifts.

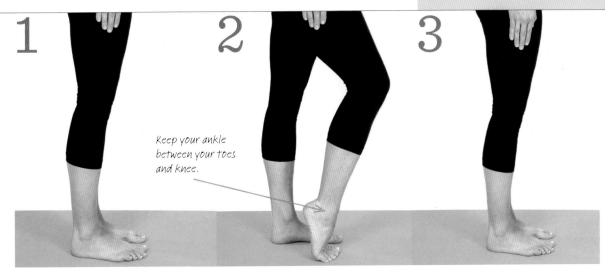

1

2

Keep your ankle between your toes and knee.

3

Stand with your feet together and your arms relaxed at your sides.

Inhale as you lift to the ball of one foot, centering your weight between your second and third toes.

Exhale as you lower your heel back down to the mat. Repeat the exercise 10 times, alternating sides.

Toe Lifts

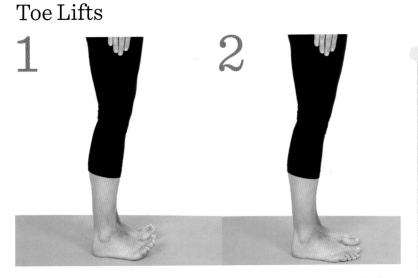

1

2

CHALLENGE YOURSELF

Press your heels together and lengthen long to grow taller as you lift your heels.

Continue to stand with your feet together and your arms relaxed at your sides. Inhale as you lift your toes, making sure everything besides your lifted toes and your foot triangles stays in the same position.

Exhale as you lower your toes back down to the mat. Repeat the exercise 10 times.

- During toe lifts, stand on one leg or close your eyes for an extra test of your balance.

- During foot rolls, lift both heels off the ground, lengthening through the top of the head, to strengthen your calves.

single-knee bends

During the single-knee bends, you do a small squat, which works your lower body and challenges your balance. As you do this exercise, keep your torso upright in the middle of your two legs as you bend. Also, pay attention to your alignment: Are your hips and shoulders squared forward? Are you keeping your ankles, knees, and hips aligned? This is a good exercise to do in front of a mirror to help you watch your alignment.

{visualize} your shoulders being stacked over your hips during the knee bends.

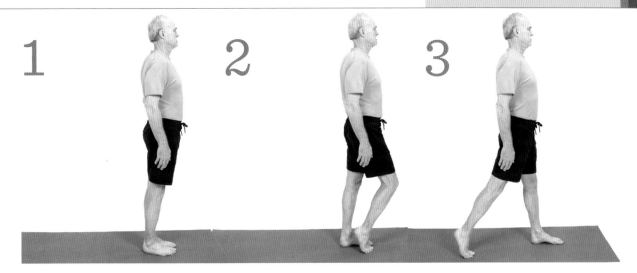

1 Stand with your feet together.

2 Inhale as you roll to the ball of your right foot.

3 Exhale as you place your right foot behind you. Bring your torso in the center between your feet to get in position to bend.

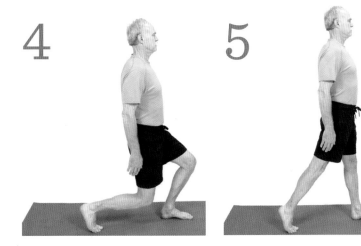

4 Inhale as you bend your knees, letting your back knee drop down toward the floor. Your shoulders should remain over your hips while your front foot stays flat on the floor.

5 Exhale as you use your core to straighten your legs. Feel the foot triangle on your left foot and the ball of the right foot press into the floor as you straighten. Repeat the knee bends 10 times before returning to starting position.

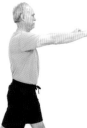

CHALLENGE YOURSELF

Position the band or pole in front of your chest or overhead.

- Hold a band or pole in front of your chest or overhead to further challenge your balance and work your upper body.

- Touch your back knee to the floor for more lower-body work.

SINGLE-KNEE BENDS

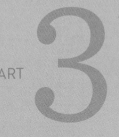

PART **3**

Pilates Equipment Exercises

Welcome to the equipment portion of the book, where each chapter includes a few exercises using a certain type of equipment. These pieces of equipment may already be in your home or can be found at many fitness centers. If you don't have any of these equipment options available but would like to purchase them, the following pages include a few ideas on what to consider in your search. Also, I have included ideas on equipment substitutes to use for the exercises at the start of the ring, arm weights, and band/pole chapters. You'll find some of my suggestions are inexpensive and readily available in your home!

finding equipment

The following are some of my recommendations for the equipment used in this part. What I share is by no means extensive when it comes to the products available, but I hope it will help you evaluate what to get as you purchase home equipment. Personally, I have purchased most of the equipment in my home from a company called Balanced Body (pilates.com), one of the leaders in manufacturing Pilates equipment and in the education of Pilates teachers.

Ring

The Pilates ring can sometimes be found in retail stores, but it is most readily available online. There are rings made of different materials, weights, and resistances. The rings that I have found most loyal to Joseph Pilates' ring design are the Spring Circles made by Balanced Body, which you can find at the website mentioned earlier. These rings come in two bands, three bands, and four bands of metal corresponding to light, medium, and heavy resistance. For the exercises in this book, a basic un-weighted, medium-resistance ring is sufficient.

Arm Weights

Small arm weights can found in many retail stores. In addition to the weights which you can hold in your hand, there are also weighted gloves and wrist weights. The wrist weights and gloves are nice, as you don't have to hold onto anything; however, it does take time to put on and take off the weights. As long as you are using a light weight of 2 to 3 pounds (1 to 1.25 kg), what kind you use is your preference.

Band or Pole

There are different materials and weights of bands and poles available. One consideration in your purchase should be how easy the band or pole is to clean, as some are easier to clean than others. I would recommend using a nonweighted pole for exercises in this part. You can also use a basic yoga strap, which is available in the fitness aisle of retail stores.

Don't feel like you have to go out and buy one of these, either; you can make your own. For example, I made the pole used in this book years ago with a basic wooden dowel rod from a local hardware store and placed rubber tips on the ends of the dowel. The rubber tips are what would be found on the bottom of a chair leg. For a few dollars, I had a great piece of equipment which clients and I have enjoyed for years.

Large Ball

When selecting a ball, an important consideration is the size. Balanced Body offers general fitness balls, including latex-free balls of various sizes. The size of the ball can be adjusted based on how much the ball is inflated. Deflating a ball slightly makes it a little smaller, while fully inflating it makes the ball larger.

Because large stability balls are used by the general fitness community, they are available through a large number of retailers. Wherever you purchase a ball, check to see if it comes with a pump. Otherwise, you will need to purchase or have access to an air pump.

Foam Roller

Foam rollers are available in different densities, sizes, and colors. If you are someone who feels more comfortable on a thicker, softer mat or bruises easily, I recommend the soft foam roller. If you enjoy a thinner mat, the firm foam roller is more appropriate. Having used several foam rollers, my personal favorite is made from a material called EVA foam. In terms of softness, I feel the EVA foam rollers are between the soft and firm roller.

As you search, you may find rollers with projections on them. Although the foam rollers with grids or projections (like the rumble roller) can be great for self-massage, they should not be used for the exercises presented in this book. Stay with a foam roller that has a smooth surface. In terms of length, a 36-inch (91.5-cm) foam roller offers the most versatility; however, a short roller can suffice for the exercises found in this book.

CHAPTER 10

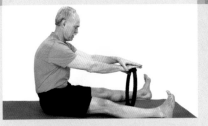

The Ring

This chapter is about exercises using the ring, which allows your body to make small, isolated movements. Even if the ring doesn't move as you press in or pull out on it, your muscles are still working isometrically. Isometric contractions are where your muscle is active but not changing length. You use isometric contractions in daily life when you carry an object or hold postures.

If you don't have a ring, you could use a small rubber ball as a substitute for some of the exercises. A rubber ball will allow you to do the exercises that require you to press in on the ring, but you'll need to omit the parts that require you to pull out on the ring.

press and pull

The press and pull is a great workout for your back and upper body. During the arm work for this exercise, you hold the ring in a number of different positions as you press in and pull out on it. As you do this, notice how the presses and pulls are more difficult when the ring is held with straight arms.

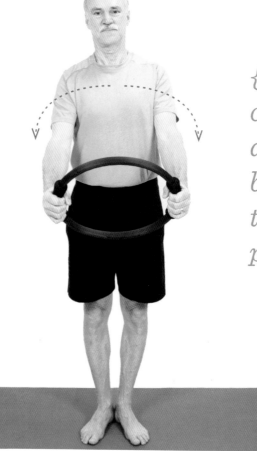

{visualize} your chest staying open and your shoulders broad as you do the ring press and pulls.

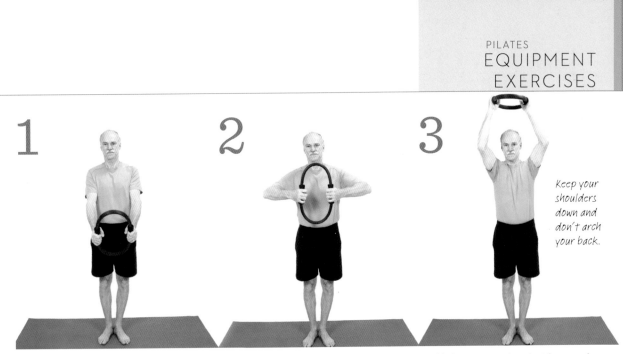

Keep your shoulders down and don't arch your back.

1 Bring the ring in front of your chest with your arms straight. Inhale as you press in on the ring. Exhale as you pull out on the ring. Repeat 10 times.

2 Hold the ring in front of your chest with your elbows bent to the sides. Inhale as you press in on the ring. Exhale as you pull out on the ring. Repeat 10 times.

3 Hold the ring overhead with your elbows slightly bent. Inhale as you press in on the ring. Exhale as you pull out on the ring. Repeat 10 times.

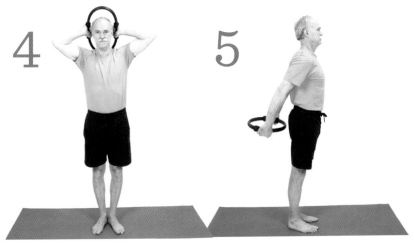

4 Hold the ring behind your head with your elbows bent to the sides. Inhale as you press in on the ring. Exhale as you pull out on the ring. Repeat 10 times.

5 Hold the ring behind your hips with your arms straight. Inhale as you press in on the ring. Exhale as you pull out on the ring. Repeat 10 times. Return to starting position.

PRESS AND PULL

bicep press and side-arm press

For the bicep press, you bend and straighten your elbow while using the ring for resistance; during the side-arm press, you try to press your entire arm into the ring toward the mat. If you place your free hand under your armpit during both exercises, you should feel the muscles in the front and back of your armpit equally engage and relax on the working arm.

BENEFITS

Strengthens the upper body

Develops the postural muscles

Connects breath to movement

{visualize} sitting tall with your shoulders stacked over your hips.

Bicep Press

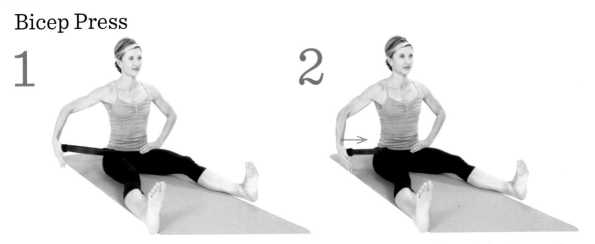

1
Sit tall with your feet open in a small V-position. Place the ring up against the side of your pelvis, making sure it's not on your waist. Your arm should be bent with your elbow facing behind you.

2
Inhale as you press in on the ring by bending your elbow. Exhale as you slowly release the press. Repeat the exercise 10 times with each of your arms.

Side-Arm Press

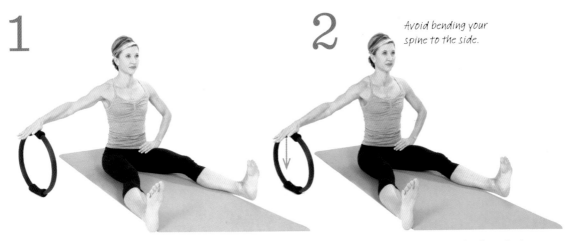

Avoid bending your spine to the side.

1
Place the ring to the side with the ring about a foot in front of your shoulder. Straighten your arm, placing your hand on the ring.

2
Inhale as you press the ring into the floor, feeling your shoulder blade slide down your back. Use your core to stay sitting up tall. Exhale as you slowly release the press on the ring. Repeat the exercise 10 times with each arm.

spine stretch

The spine stretch with the ring adds some greater abdominal work to the spine stretch on the mat. As you perform this, pay attention so the ring presses down from your abdominals instead of your arms. If you'd like to add an extra stretch, flex and point your feet during the exercise.

Strengthens the abdominals

Develops spine articulation and control

Improves spine flexibility

{visualize} the press of the ring initiating from your abdominals.

1

2

3

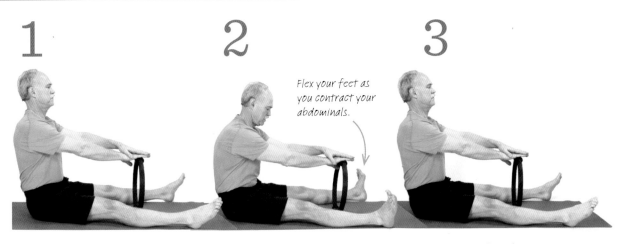

Flex your feet as you contract your abdominals.

Sit tall with your legs in a small V and your feet pointed. Place the ring upright in front with your hands on top of the ring.

Inhale as you lengthen through your spine to prepare. Exhale as you contract your abdominals, bringing your spine into a deep scoop to a C-shape.

Inhale as you lengthen your spine back to sitting, articulating one bone of your spine at a time. Point your feet as you grow tall to return to starting position. Repeat the exercise 10 times.

MAKE IT EASIER

Bend your knees for less of a stretch to the back of your legs.

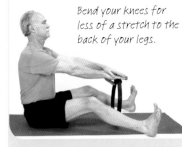

- Sit on blocks or bend your knees to help you more easily sit tall.
- Return to the spine stretch on the mat without the ring for less abdominal work.

CHALLENGE YOURSELF

Lift one arm off of the ring, keeping your shoulders square.

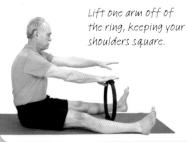

Do the spine stretch with one arm on the ring for an extra challenge to your upper body and core.

SPINE STRETCH

inner thigh presses and glute pulls

During the inner thigh presses and glute pulls, you stabilize the ring with your bottom leg. To get into position, place the ring to the front edge of your mat so the ring is slightly in front of your body and then place your bottom leg in the ring. You then align your spine in a side-lying position in the center of the mat and position your top leg.

BENEFITS

Strengthens the inner thighs

Strengthens the outer glutes

Develops core stabilization

{visualize} your top leg lengthening long to help engage your core.

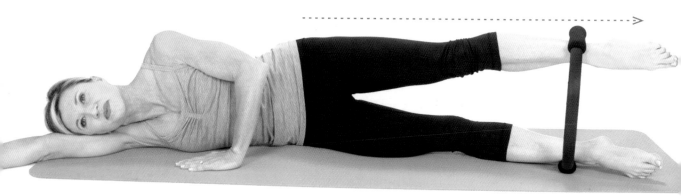

Inner Thigh Presses

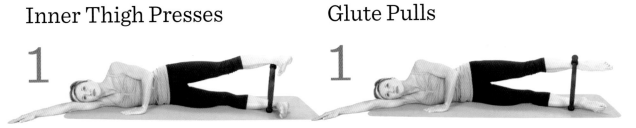

1

Lie on your side with your bottom leg inside the ring and your top leg on top of the ring.

2

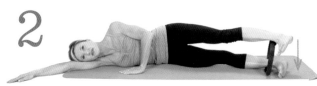

Inhale as you press your leg toward the mat using your inner thighs.

3

Exhale as you slowly release the press on the ring. Repeat the exercise 10 times.

Glute Pulls

1

Continuing to lie on your side on the mat with your bottom leg inside the ring, bring your top leg inside the ring.

Hold the ring stable with your bottom leg.

2

Inhale as you pull up on the ring, using your outer glutes to pull.

3

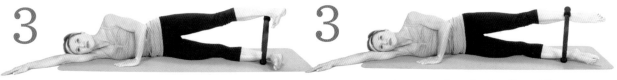

Exhale as you release to pull on the ring. Repeat the exercise 10 times. Repeat both exercises on the other side.

side-lying leg work

During the side-lying leg work, you press on the ring, release the press, lift your leg up to the ceiling, and lower your leg to the ring. The press on the ring works your inner thigh, while the leg lift works your outer glutes. Throughout the entire sequence, keep your top leg lengthened long.

BENEFITS

Strengthens the inner thighs and outer glutes

Develops core stabilization

Requires coordination

{visualize} releasing the ring slowly so it's still and steady as you lift your leg.

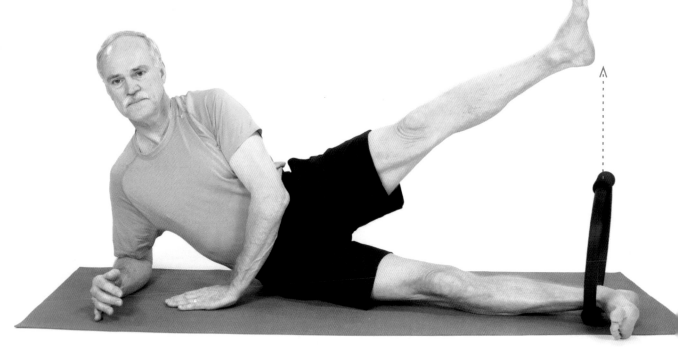

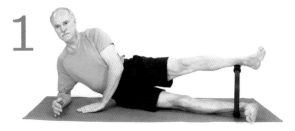

1 Come up on your elbow in the center of the mat with your ribcage lifted and your bottom leg inside the ring. Place the ring about a foot in front of your torso with your top leg on top of the ring.

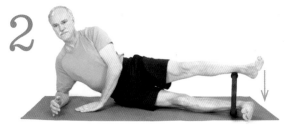

2 Inhale as you press the ring into the mat with your top leg by using your inner thighs.

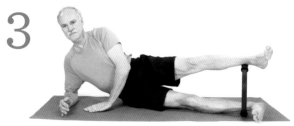

3 Exhale as you slowly release the ring, doing so slowly enough that the ring is still during the next step.

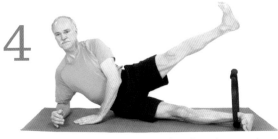

4 Inhale as you lift your leg to the ceiling, keeping your leg lengthened long.

MAKE IT EASIER

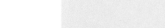

Lie flat on your side.

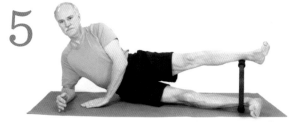

5 Exhale as you lower your leg back to the ring. Repeat the exercise 10 times before repeating on the other side.

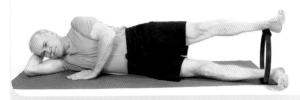

- Lie on your side for an easier upper-body position.
- Return to practicing the inner thigh presses and glute pulls found in this chapter for an exercise that uses less hip range of motion and allows you to better keep the ring stable.

butt blasters

The butt blasters use the ring to work the back of your legs and glutes. Because you hold your thighs lifted as you bend and straighten your knees, you will be using your hamstrings and glutes independently of one another. Keep your thigh lift small and your abdominals engaged to protect your back, and stop if you have any back tension.

{visualize} your glutes squeezing together as you lift your thighs.

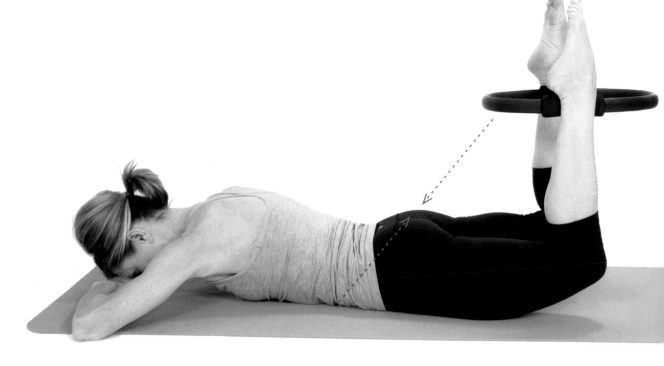

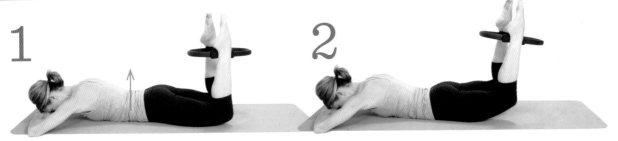

1 Lie on your stomach with your navel drawn up and away from the mat. Rest your head on your hands with your palms flat on the floor. Bend your knees at a 90-degree angle with the ring between your ankles.

2 Inhale as you lift your thighs slightly off the mat, squeezing your glutes and keeping your abdominals engaged.

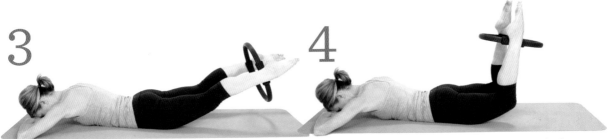

3 Exhale as you straighten your knees while keeping your thighs lifted.

4 Inhale as you bend your knees, still keeping your thighs lifted.

MAKE IT EASIER

Do the exercise with one leg at a time.

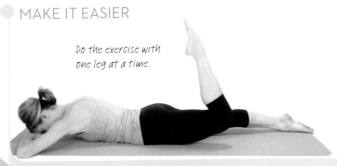

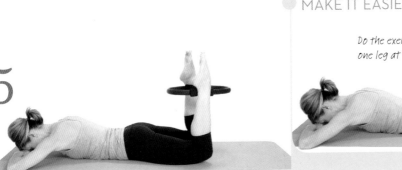

5 Once your knees are bent at a 90-degree angle, exhale as you lower your thighs back to the mat. Repeat the exercise 10 times.

- Do this exercise without the ring with one of your legs at a time for less work for your legs and core.
- Practice just the thigh lift or the knee straightening and bending until you're strong enough to do the full exercise.

ab work with ring in hands

The ab work with ring in hands can add upper-body strengthening to the mat work exercises you do on your back. Here, I show you how to do the double-leg stretch with the ring.

{visualize} long arms with the length extending through your fingertips.

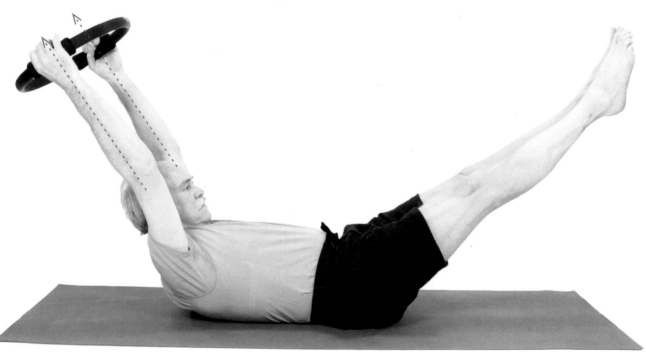

1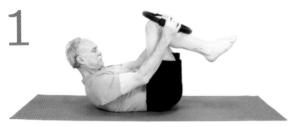

Lie flat on your back. Pull both knees to your chest and lift your head, neck, and shoulders. Place your hands on the ring with the ring over your shins.

2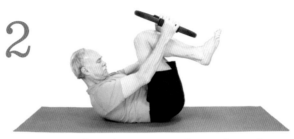

Inhale as you pull your knees to your chest and press in on the ring.

3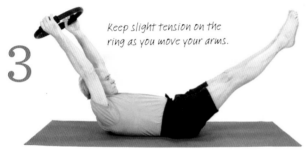

Keep slight tension on the ring as you move your arms.

Exhale as you extend your legs long at a 45-degree angle as your arms reach long to the ceiling and overhead, if possible.

4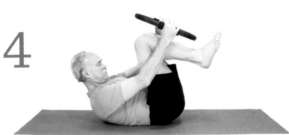

Inhale as you pull your knees back to your chest. Repeat 10 times. Return to starting position.

CHALLENGE YOURSELF

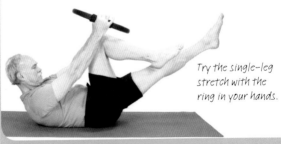

Try the single-leg stretch with the ring in your hands.

- Do other abdominal exercises with the ring to give yourself more of an upper-body challenge.
- Add a pullout on the ring while the ring is overhead for more upper-body work.

CHAPTER 11

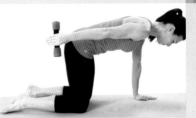

Arm Weights

This chapter contains various upper-body exercises that can be done as you hold light arm weights. Using weights will help improve your upper-body strength and endurance. I would recommend starting with weights of 2 or 3 pounds (1 or 1.25 kg). You could also use a light object that can be easily gripped as a substitute for arm weights, such as a full plastic water bottle.

If you don't have weights on hand when doing any of these exercises, feel free to do them by simply keeping your fingers long.

hug a tree

Hug a tree works the muscles of your midback, shoulders, and chest, while the addition of arm weights challenges the muscles of your chest, tops of your arms, and upper back. As you close your arms on an inhalation, your shoulder blades slide apart and the back of your ribcage can open and expand. On the exhalation, feel your shoulder blades slide together and squeeze the air out of your lungs.

BENEFITS

Improves breath control

Strengthens the upper body

Develops shoulder blade mobility

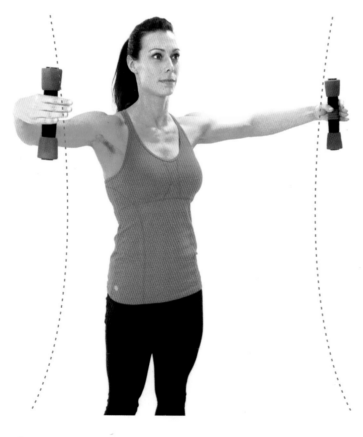

{visualize} your- self rounding your arms as if hugging a big tree.

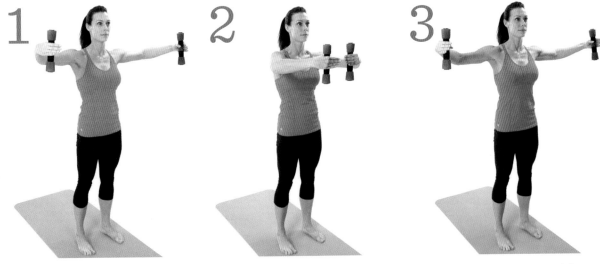

1 Stand with your arms at shoulder height. Hold the arm weights with your palms facing forward and elbows facing back.

2 Inhale as you draw your arms together, as if hugging a big tree.

3 Exhale as you open your arms, sliding your shoulder blades together in back. Keep your elbows going to the back of the room.

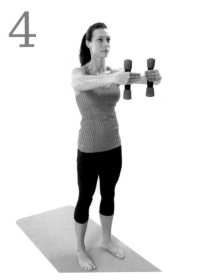

4 Repeat the exercise 10 times. Repeat 10 more times with reverse breathing, exhaling as you close your arms in front of you and inhaling as you open your arms to the side.

MAKE IT EASIER

Hold your fingers long as you do the exercise without arm weights.

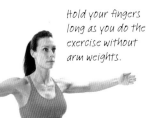

- Perform this exercise without arm weights while standing for less of an upper-body challenge.

- Do this exercise without arm weights while lying on your back to lessen the work on the top of your arms.

HUG A TREE

rowing 1

During rowing 1, your torso and spine stay stable as you move your arms, making this a great workout for your shoulders. The addition of arm weights to the large arm movements strengthens the muscles of your arms, shoulders, and midback. When doing this exercise, stay within a motion where you can keep your shoulders down to help ensure the work is staying in your arms and midback.

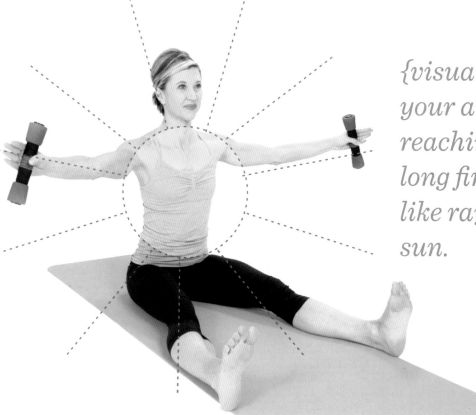

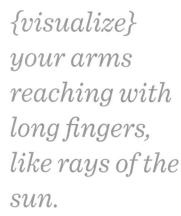

{visualize}
your arms
reaching with
long fingers,
like rays of the
sun.

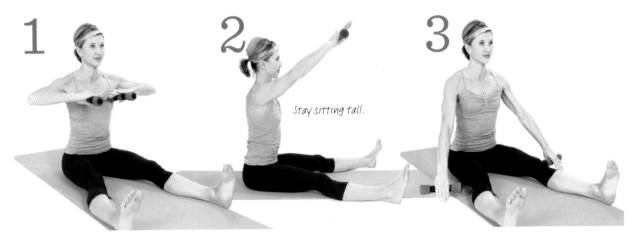

1

Sit on the mat with your legs in a small V-position, if possible. Holding the arm weights, place your thumbs near your armpits and bring your elbows out to your sides.

2

Stay sitting tall.

Inhale as you stretch your arms to the ceiling at a 45-degree angle.

3

Exhale as you lower your fingertips to the ground, keeping your chest open to avoid rounding your shoulders forward.

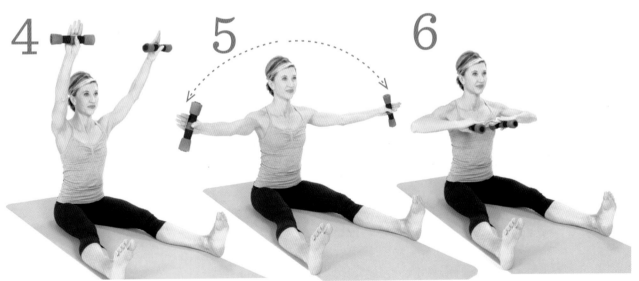

4

After your fingers touch the ground, lift your arms overhead as you inhale.

5

On a long exhale, draw a large semi-circle with each of your arms.

6

Continue the long exhale as you return to starting position. Repeat the exercise 10 times.

rowing 2

Rowing 2 works your shoulders, midback, and spine. It has similar arm motions to rowing 1 but adds movement for your torso and spine. The forward rounding and hinge of your spine at an angle with the arm weights is a great strengthener for your midback. When lengthening to a forward hinge, start at your tailbone and grow tall through the top of your head.

{visualize} your arms and torso moving as a unit as you go from a forward hinge to sitting.

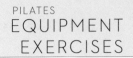
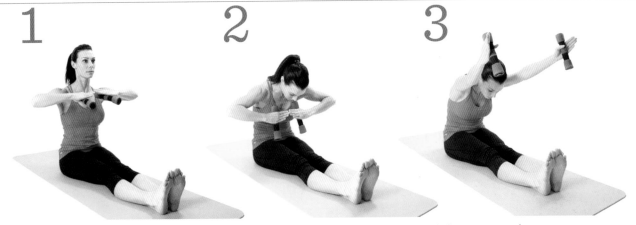

1

Sit on the mat with your legs together and straight, if possible. Holding the arm weights, place your thumbs near your armpits and bring your elbows out to your sides.

2

Round forward, keeping your abdominals scooped, as you inhale.

3

Exhale as you stretch your arms overhead.

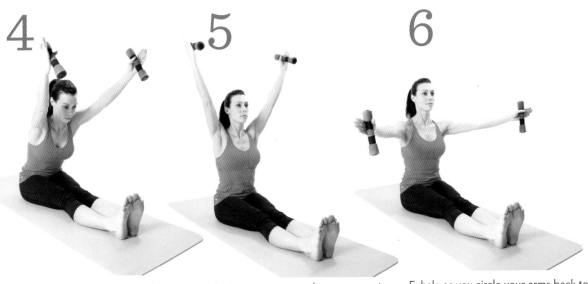

4

Inhale as you grow your spine long at a 45-degree angle over your legs, if your flexibility allows. Lengthen by pressing your tailbone behind you and growing through the rest of your spine.

5

Moving your arms and torso as a unit, exhale as you bring your arms and torso to an upright position. Inhale as you lengthen long through your spine, holding your arms overhead.

6

Exhale as you circle your arms back to starting position. Repeat the exercise 10 times.

ROWING 2

arm circles

Although this exercise is called *arm circles*, your arms do not make a true circle; instead, your arms make more a triangular pattern. The movement of your arms in the natural range of your shoulder joints makes this a good exercise for your shoulder joints' range of motion. As you use your arm weights, feel the movement originating from your midback between your shoulder blades as you strengthen your upper body.

{visualize} the motion of your arms drawing triangular patterns like pieces of pie.

1

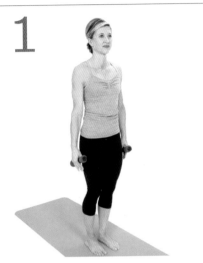

Holding arm weights, stand with your arms down at the sides of your body and your palms turned to face your body.

2

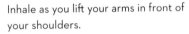

Inhale as you lift your arms in front of your shoulders.

3

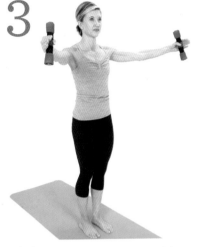

Exhale as you open your arms out to a V-position, keeping your arms in your peripheral vision to stay within the natural range of your shoulder joints.

4

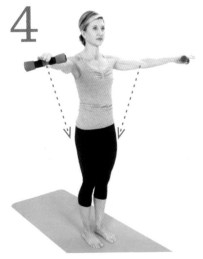

Continue a long exhale as you draw your arms down toward your hips with your palms facing your body. After 10 repetitions, reverse the direction of the circle and do 10 more repetitions. Return to starting position.

MAKE IT EASIER

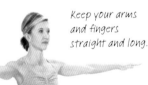

Keep your arms and fingers straight and long.

- Do this exercise without arm weights while standing for less of an upper-body challenge.

- Do this exercise without weights while on your back on the mat for even less work for your upper body.

ARM CIRCLES

serve a tray

Serve a tray is a nice workout for your arms and midback, which are further challenged by the addition of arm weights. During this exercise, keep your palms up to the ceiling and have your gaze follow the arm motions. You should feel the opposing slide of your shoulder blades down your back as your arms stretch at an angle toward the ceiling.

{visualize} yourself lifting a large tray or ball up to the ceiling at an angle.

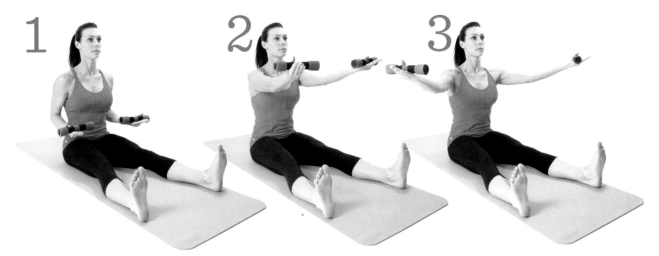

1 Sit with your elbows touching the sides of your ribcage. Hold the arm weights palms up.

2 Inhale as you stretch your arms up to the ceiling at a slight angle.

3 Keeping your arms lifted, exhale as you open your arms to a small V-position.

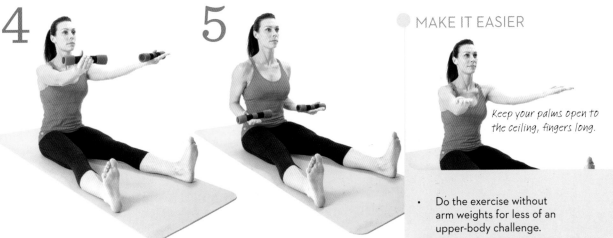

4 Inhale as you return your arms back to shoulder-distance apart.

5 Exhale as you bend your arms back to starting position. Repeat this exercise 10 times.

MAKE IT EASIER

Keep your palms open to the ceiling, fingers long.

- Do the exercise without arm weights for less of an upper-body challenge.

- Perform the exercise sitting on a chair or standing for easier lower-body and torso positioning.

SERVE A TRAY

shaving

Shaving works not only the muscles of your arms (such as the triceps), but also works the muscles deep into your midback with the overhead movement. The addition of arm weights makes for even deeper work. This exercise requires a great deal of shoulder flexibility to be done correctly; be careful to feel the work in your midback and to keep your shoulders down to avoid tension in your neck.

BENEFITS

- Strengthens the arms and midback
- Prepares the body to do work overhead
- Develops shoulder blade control

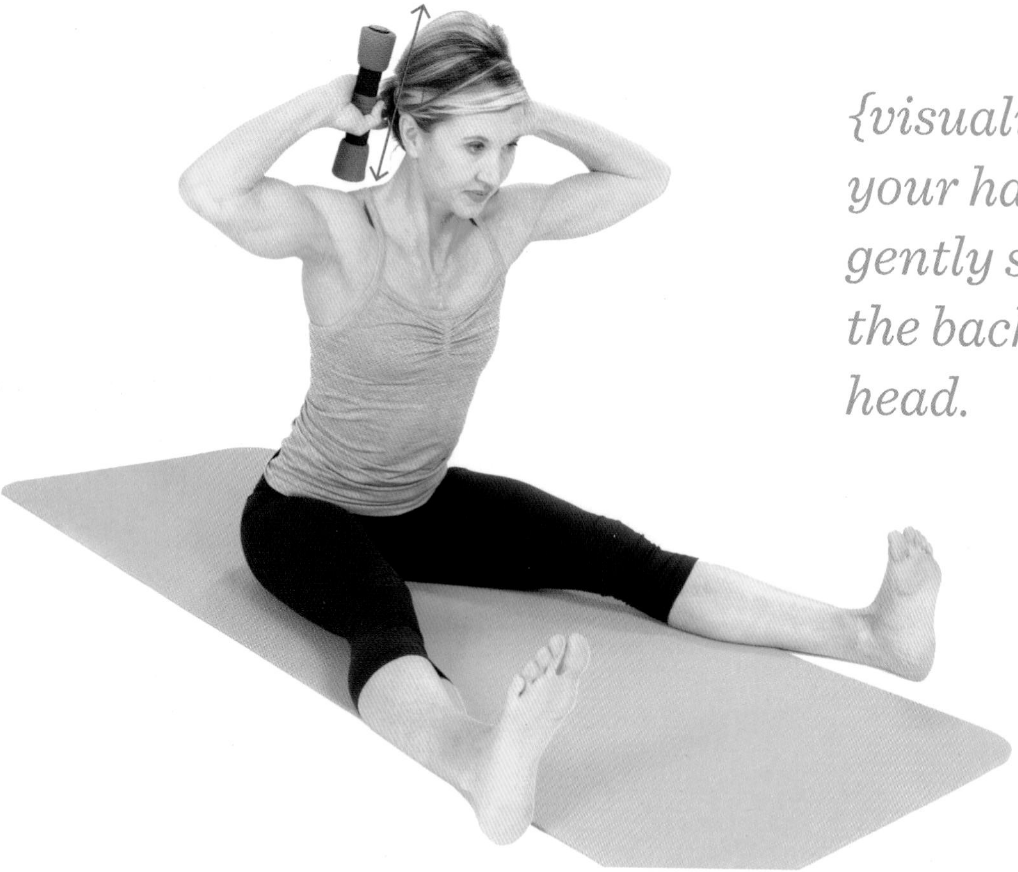

{visualize} your hands gently shaving the back of your head.

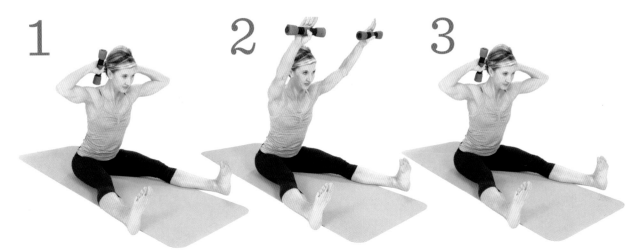

1
Holding arm weights, sit with your hands behind your head and your elbows at the sides of your body.

2
Inhale as you extend your arms at about a 70-degree diagonal up to the ceiling, keeping your shoulder blades down and away from your ears.

3
Exhale as you bend your arms behind your head to return to starting position. Repeat the exercise 10 times.

MAKE IT EASIER

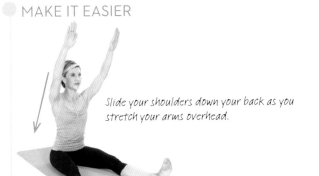

Slide your shoulders down your back as you stretch your arms overhead.

- Do shaving without arm weights for less of an upper-body challenge.
- Perform the shaving motion with your hands coming in front of your face instead of behind your head for an easier shoulder position.
- Do the exercise sitting on a chair or in less of a forward hinge for an easier lower-body position to sit tall.

CHALLENGE YOURSELF

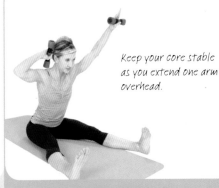

Keep your core stable as you extend one arm overhead.

Perform single-arm shaving, alternating arms, to challenge your core stability.

SHAVING

pullbacks and tricep extension

Both the pullbacks and tricep extensions work muscles in the back of your arms and midback. Doing these two exercises when on all fours allows gravity to add resistance to the motion, in addition to the extra challenge from the arm weights. Be careful to keep both your shoulders and your hips stable throughout the exercises.

{visualize} your shoulders staying level as you keep them and your hips square.

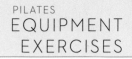

Pullbacks

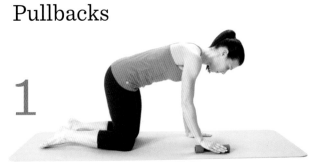

1 Kneel on all fours with an arm weight in one of your hands, keeping your head in line with your spine and your spine straight.

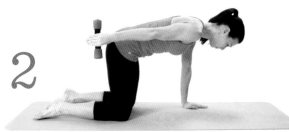

2 Inhale as you lift your arm with the weight up to the ceiling next to your hip.

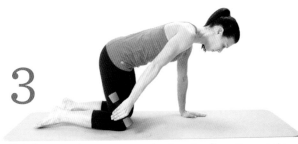

3 Exhale as you lower your arm back to the floor. Repeat this exercise 10 times before returning to starting position.

Tricep Extensions

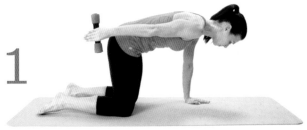

1 Continue to kneel on all fours with an arm weight in one of your hands. Have your arm at the side of your body.

Only your forearm and hand should be moving.

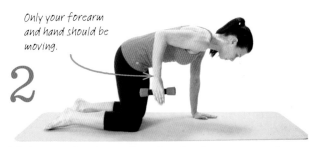

2 Inhale as you bend your elbow, keeping the upper part of your arm still.

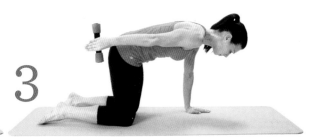

3 Exhale as you straighten your elbow. Repeat this exercise 10 times, continuing to keep your shoulders and hips square, before returning to starting position.

CHAPTER 12

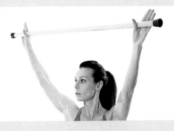

Band or Pole

The exercises in this chapter strengthen and warm up your upper body and midback using a resistance band or pole. Holding one of these will help you stay symmetrical and guide your upper-body movements during the exercises.

An object that is light and long enough for your arms to be in a wide V-position can be used for these exercises. Appropriate alternatives for a band or pole include a long broom, rope, strap, or belt. Or if you are a golfer, a long golf club is a great alternative!

front arm lifts

Front arm lifts move your shoulder gently through the range of the shoulder joint as you hold a band or pole. Because this exercise activates the muscles of your shoulder and midback, you can use it as a warm-up before other pole and band work exercises. As you move your arms, keep your core engaged to avoid arching your back or elevating your shoulders as you bring your arms overhead.

BENEFITS

Warms up the shoulder joint

Teaches upper-body control

Activates the muscles of the shoulders and midback

{visualize} a pivot point at your shoulders as you bring your arms overhead.

1

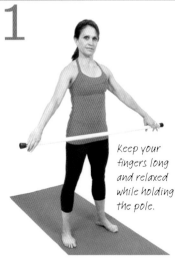

Keep your fingers long and relaxed while holding the pole.

Stand with your feet hip-distance apart. Let the pole rest naturally in front of you at hip level, arms straight and fingers long.

2

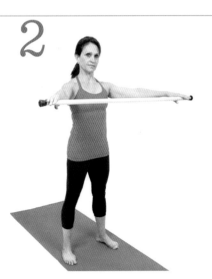

Inhale as you lift the pole to the front of your chest, keeping your arms straight.

3

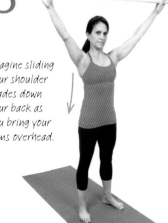

Imagine sliding your shoulder blades down your back as you bring your arms overhead.

Exhale as you lift the pole overhead, being careful to avoid arching your back. At the top, your arms should be symmetrical and your head should be in the center underneath the pole.

4

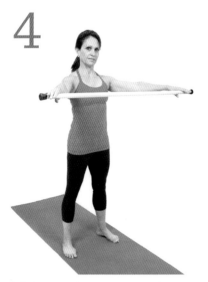

Inhale as you lower your straight arms in front of your chest.

5

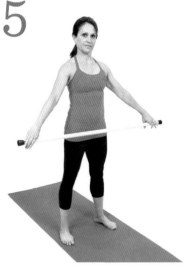

Exhale as you lower the pole down to your hips. Repeat the exercise 10 times.

MAKE IT EASIER

Keep your shoulders wide and your arms straight.

- Lift your arms to the front of your chest and down, skipping the overhead lift for less shoulder range of motion.

- Lie on your back on the floor during the exercise to lessen the weight of your arms.

overhead arm press

The overhead arm press strengthens the muscles of your midback as you hold up the weight of your arms against gravity with a band or pole. As you do this exercise, move with intention, feeling the opposing reach of your fingers upward and your shoulders downward as you press your arms overhead. Keeping your shoulders down helps concentrate the work to your midback instead of tensing your neck.

BENEFITS

Develops postural muscles

Strengthens the shoulders and mid-back

Teaches upper-body symmetry

{visualize} your fingers reaching long to the ceiling while your shoulder blades slide down your back.

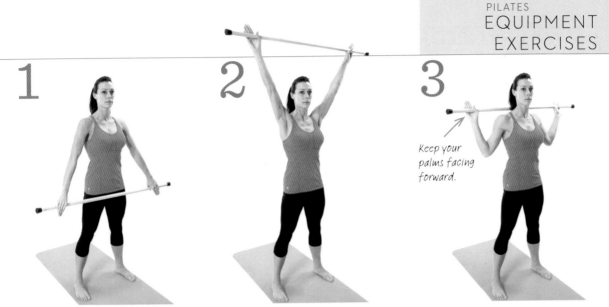

1 Stand with your feet hip-distance apart. Let the pole rest naturally in front of you at hip level, arms straight and fingers long.

2 Inhale as you bring the pole in front of your chest. Exhale as you lift the pole overhead.

3 Inhale as you bend your elbows to your ribcage and lower the pole behind your head.

Keep your palms facing forward.

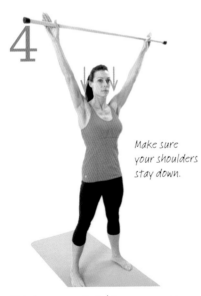

Make sure your shoulders stay down.

4 Exhale as you straighten your arms overhead, engaging the muscles between your shoulder blades to press your arms to the ceiling. Repeat steps 3 and 4 10 times before returning to starting position.

CHALLENGE YOURSELF

Keep your shoulders down as you hold your arms overhead.

Do single-arm presses overhead by bending one of your elbows to your ribcage on the inhale and straightening on the exhale for 10 repetitions, holding your non-moving arm still and steady overhead for work on your endurance. Repeat with your other arm.

OVERHEAD ARM PRESS

front arm press

The front arm press strengthens the muscles on the top of your shoulder while the band or pole helps you keep symmetical. For this exercise, pay attention to the alignment of your wrists, elbows, and shoulders to practice proper technique; they should remain parallel to the floor. If you are looking forward in a mirror, your elbows should be hidden behind the pole or band.

{visualize} your arms gliding on top of a level surface in order to keep your wrists, elbows, and shoulders level.

1

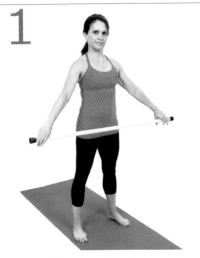

Stand with your feet hip-distance apart. Let the pole rest naturally in front of you at hip level, arms straight and fingers long.

2

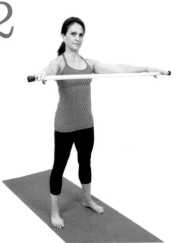

Inhale as you lift the pole in front of your chest. Exhale while holding the pole in front of your chest.

3

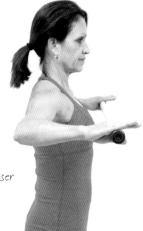

Slide your shoulder blades closer together.

Inhale as you bend your arms, bringing the pole closer to the center of your chest and keeping your elbows lifted the same height from the ground.

4

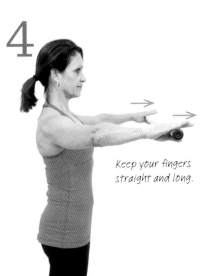

Keep your fingers straight and long.

Exhale as you straighten your arms forward. Repeat steps 3 and 4 10 times before returning to starting position.

CHALLENGE YOURSELF

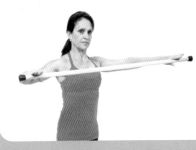

Do single front arm presses by bending one of your elbows on the inhale and straightening on the exhale for 10 repetitions, holding your nonmoving arm still and steady in front to work on your endurance. Repeat with your other arm.

behind-the-back arm bends

Behind-the-back arm bends stretch your chest and shoulders while gently strengthening the muscles of your midback. The more you reach the band or pole behind your body, the greater the chest opening and stretch. This is a beneficial exercise to work on the flexibility needed for athletics.

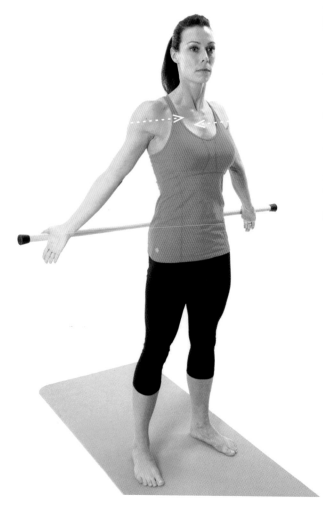

{visualize} your shoulder blades sliding closer to your spine as your chest stretches.

1

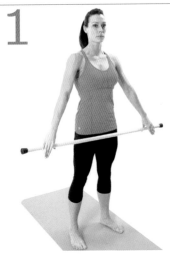

Stand with your feet hip-distance apart. Let the pole rest naturally in front of you at hip level, arms straight and fingers long.

2

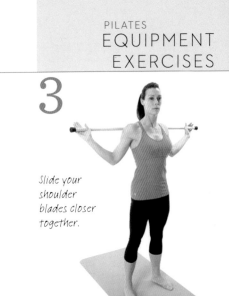

Inhale as you bring the pole in front of your chest. Exhale as you lift the pole overhead.

3

Slide your shoulder blades closer together.

Inhale as you bend your elbows to your waist, lowering the pole behind your head.

4

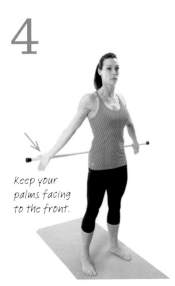

Keep your palms facing to the front.

Exhale as you straighten your elbows toward the floor with your arms still behind you.

5

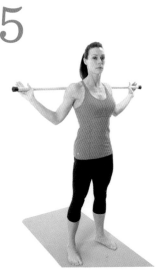

Inhale as you bend your elbows to your waist, lifting the pole behind your back.

6

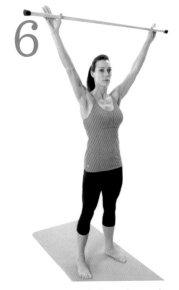

Exhale as you lift the pole overhead. Repeat steps 3 through 6 10 times before returning to starting position.

BEHIND-THE-BACK ARM BENDS

side stretch

The side stretch requires a focus on length. Instead of collapsing to the side, your torso is lengthened up and over like stretching over a ball. This lengthening stretches each side of your spine even more and puts the work into your muscles instead of stressing your joints. Holding the pole overhead allows for more of a stretch to your shoulders, sides, and back.

{visualize} both sides of your torso lengthening as you stretch to the side.

1

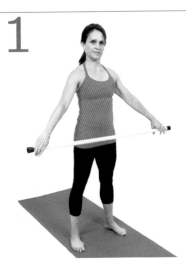

Stand with your feet hip-distance apart. Let the pole rest naturally in front of you at hip level, arms straight and fingers long.

2

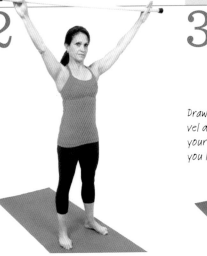

Inhale as you bring the pole in front of your chest. Exhale as you lift the pole overhead.

3

Draw your navel deeper to your spine as you lengthen.

Inhale as you lift the top of your head to the ceiling, lengthening your spine. Keeping the length to your back and spine, stretch to one side on an exhale.

4

Make sure your head is directly between your arms.

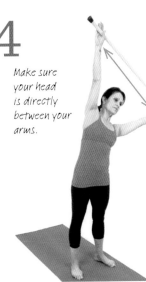

Holding the side stretch, inhale as you lengthen your torso longer to the side. Make sure you are going directly to the side.

5

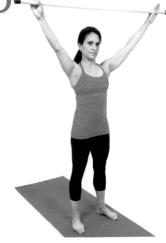

Exhale as you lift your torso back to the center. Repeat the exercise, alternating sides 10 times, before returning to starting position.

MAKE IT EASIER

Keep the length in your spine and torso.

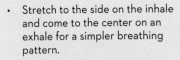

- Stretch to the side on the inhale and come to the center on an exhale for a simpler breathing pattern.

- Sit on a chair while doing this exercise to help keep your hips stable during the exercise.

SIDE STRETCH

209

torso twist

Torso twists using a band or pole to bring your arms overhead add a spiraling stretch to the muscles of your back and
arms. As you do this exercise, you work the oblique muscles
on the side of your abdomen as you rotate to each side. Keep
equal weight in each foot and your hips still during the twist
to isolate the rotation at your spine.

BENEFITS

Teaches abdominal oblique control

Develops upper-body endurance

Requires concentration to isolate
movement

Improves spinal flexibility

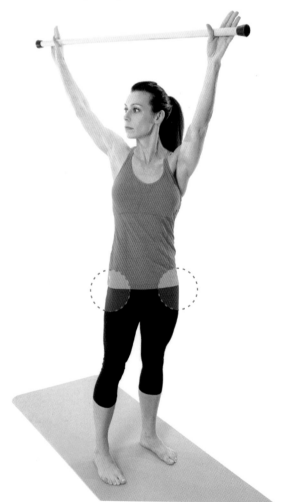

*{visualize} head-
lights on your hips
and keep them
shining forward
throughout the
twists.*

1

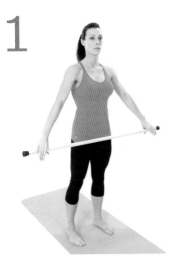

Stand with your feet hip-distance apart. Let the pole rest naturally in front of you at hip level, arms straight and fingers long.

2

Keep your shoulders down.

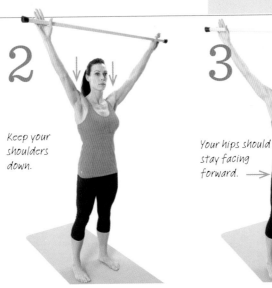

Inhale as you bring the pole in front of your chest. Exhale as you lift the pole overhead.

3

Your hips should stay facing forward.

Inhale as you rotate halfway to one side.

4

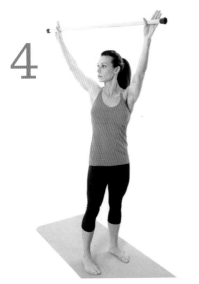

Exhale as you rotate the rest of the way to the side, only rotating as far as is comfortable for your spine. Try to focus the rotation on your midback.

5

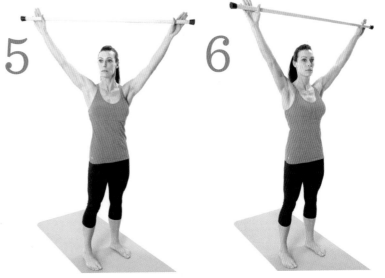

Inhale as you rotate halfway to center.

6

Exhale as you rotate back to center. Repeat the exercise to the other side. Repeat, alternating sides, 10 times.

CHAPTER 13

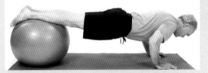

Large Ball

This chapter presents exercises you can do with a balance ball. Several of the ball exercises test your balance and aid in developing symmetry in your body. Because of the balance challenge and the fact that you are higher up from the mat, you need to be conscientious of your safety and avoid the tendency to roll.

Various sizes of balls are available. A good ball size allows your hips and knees to rest at a right angle when you sit comfortably on it. Thus, if you are more petite, you should use a smaller diameter ball; if you are taller, you need a larger ball.

bridge with arm circles

The bridge with arm circles stretches the muscles of your chest. Holding your hips lifted on the bridge uses your glutes and core muscles, which helps stabilize your ribcage. The ball helps by supporting your head and shoulders but allowing your arms to reach toward the floor during the circles for an extra stretch.

BENEFITS

Stretches the muscles of the chest

Improves shoulder flexibility

Challenges balance

Develops glute and core endurance

{visualize} your arm drawing a half-circle with each movement.

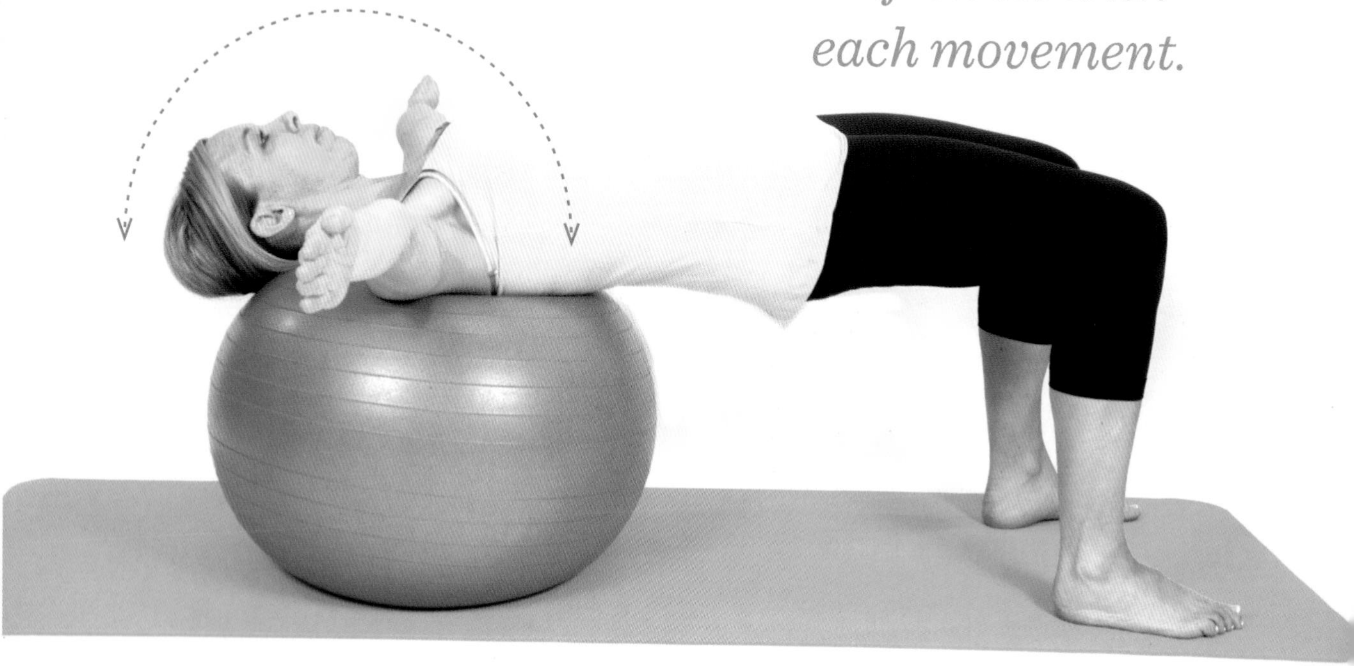

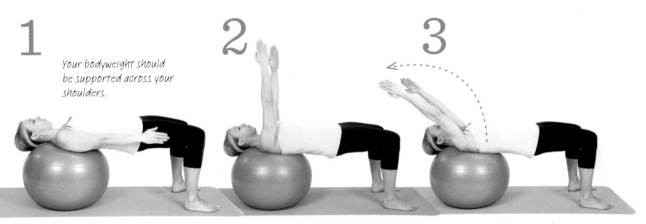

1

Your bodyweight should be supported across your shoulders.

Support your neck and shoulders on the ball. Bend your knees at a 90-degree angle. Squeeze your glutes as you hold your pelvis lifted in line with your knees and shoulders.

2

Inhale as you bring your arms over your shoulders.

3

Continue the inhale as you bring your arms overhead.

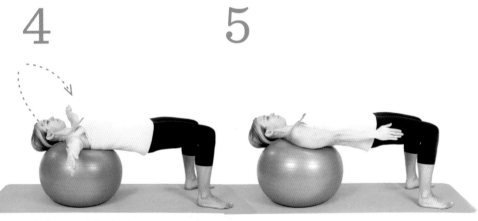

4

Exhale as you slowly draw a semicircle with each hand, bringing your arms out to your sides. Let your hands fall as close to the floor as is comfortable to stretch.

5

Finish the exhale as you return your hands to the side of your hips, completing the semicircle. Repeat the circle the same direction 5 times before reversing for the same number of repetitions. Return to starting position.

BRIDGE WITH ARM CIRCLES

bridges with feet on ball

Bridges with feet on ball provide your body with feedback on your balance during the bridge. The ball has the tendency to roll the opposite direction you are leaning, so take your time throughout the spinal roll-up and rolldown, articulating through one bone at a time.

{visualize} one bone of your spine at a time peeling off the mat on the way up and use the same control on the rolldown.

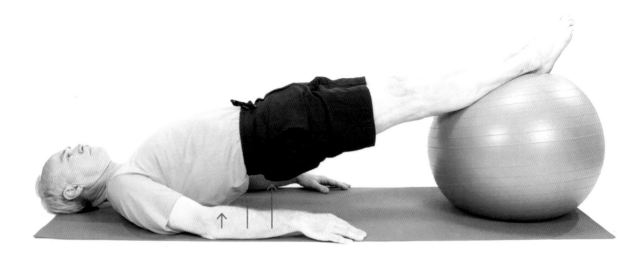

1

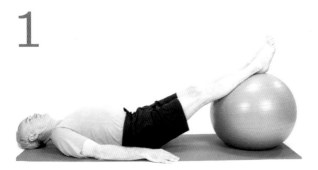

Lie on your back with your feet and calves on the ball, arms relaxed at the sides of your body.

2

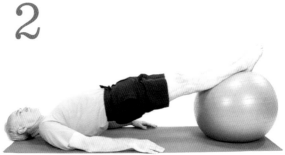

Inhale as you do a small pelvic curl, lifting your tailbone off the mat. On a long exhale, roll up through the rest of your spine one bone at a time, stopping when the weight is across your shoulders.

3

Release the pelvic tuck last to the mat.

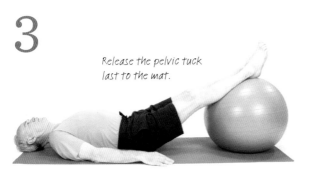

Inhale as you open your chest and place your midback on the floor. Exhale as you slowly roll the rest of your spine down to the mat. Repeat the exercise 10 times.

CHALLENGE YOURSELF

Keep your hips lifted up at the same height as you bend your knees.

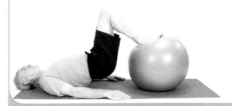

- Hold your arms up to the ceiling for more of a challenge to your balance.

- Hold the top of the bridge and bend your knees to do hamstring curls.

- Hold the bridge and do single-leg lifts to strengthen your legs and challenge your balance.

BRIDGES WITH FEET ON BALL

217

round back and round back with twist

The round back uses a pelvic curl, in which you tuck your tailbone underneath you to engage your abdominals. Use the ball to guide your curl, allowing it to roll slightly forward as you round your back. When you add the twist, keep equal weight in both legs and your pelvis. For safety during the round back exercises, sit to the front of the ball so there is plenty of room behind you on the ball.

BENEFITS

Strengthens the abdominals

Challenges balance

Develops spine articulation

Improves spine rotation

{visualize} your spine coming to a large C-shape as you round your back.

Round Back

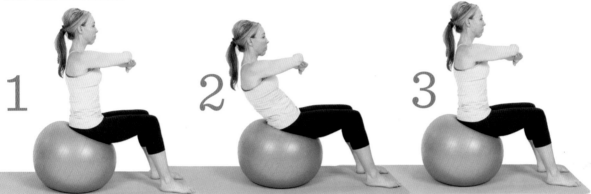

1 Sit on the ball with your feet on the floor, arms directly in front of your chest and crossed.

2 Inhale as you scoop your lower abdominals and curl your pelvis underneath you, feeling the ball move a few inches forward.

3 Exhale as you press your tailbone to the back, growing your spine long to the ceiling. Continue articulating your spine until you reach the top of your head. Repeat this exercise 10 times.

Round Back with Twist

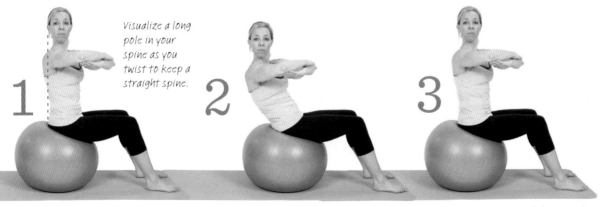

Visualize a long pole in your spine as you twist to keep a straight spine.

1 Continue to sit on the ball with your feet on the floor, arms directly in front of your chest and crossed. Inhale as you rotate your spine to one side.

2 Exhale as you round back, staying in the rotated position.

3 Inhale as you come out of the round back position and return to the rotated position. Exhale as you rotate your torso back to center. Repeat this exercise 10 times, alternating sides.

shoulder slides and plank push-ups

More than just a push-up, the shoulder slides and plank push-ups strengthen your arms and challenge your balance. Balancing on the ball helps ensure you are getting equal effort from each of your arms. As you do this exercise, recognize how the position of the ball under your legs changes the intensity of the work.

BENEFITS

Strengthens the muscles of the arms

Strengthens the muscles of the back and core

Challenges balance

{visualize} your shoulder blades staying stable on your back throughout the push-up circle.

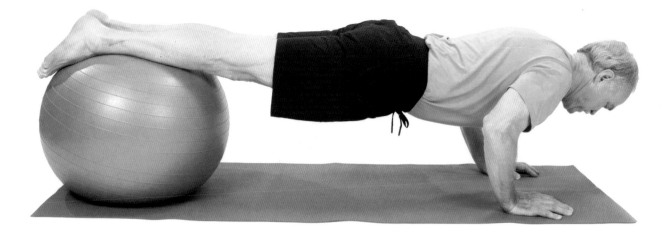

Shoulder Slides

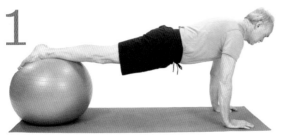

Come to a plank with the ball underneath your legs. Place your palms on the floor, fingers facing away from your body.

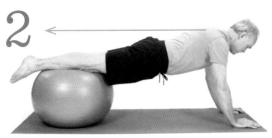

Inhale as you push your body away from your hands, hinging at your shoulders.

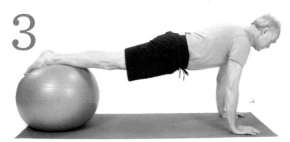

Exhale as you pull your shoulders back over your hands. Repeat this exercise 10 times.

Plank Push-Ups

Have your elbows touch the sides of your ribcage as they bend.

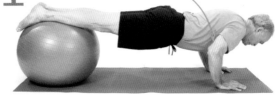

In a plank position with the ball underneath your legs, inhale as you bend your elbows and lower your face toward the floor.

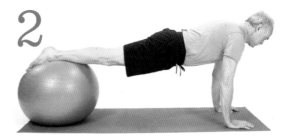

Exhale as you straighten your arms, keeping your shoulders above your wrists. Repeat the exercise 10 times.

CHALLENGE YOURSELF

- Have the ball closer to your feet for more of a challenge to your core and arms.
- Hold one leg to the ceiling for an intense challenge to your balance.

side lifts

Side lifts are a great exercise for your torso. To work the correct muscles, you want to try for a straight line from your ankle, knee, hip, shoulders, and head through the entire lift. Finishing with a long stretch over the ball gives an extra workout to those muscles.

BENEFITS

Challenges balance

Strengthens the oblique abdominal and back muscles

Improves spinal flexibility

{visualize} your body enclosed between two walls to keep your body in a straight position.

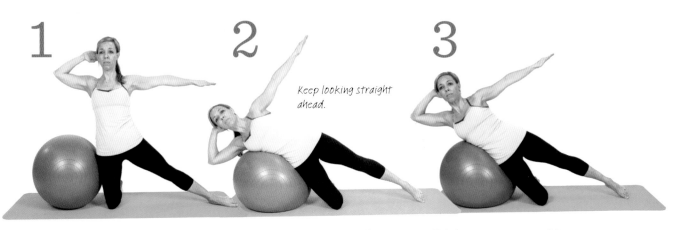

1

Kneel next to the ball with the side of your hip on the ball. Extend your leg farthest from the ball long and out to the side, and place the opposite hand behind your head.

2

Keep looking straight ahead.

Inhale as you stretch your side over the ball.

3

Exhale as you use your oblique abdominal muscles to lift your upper torso off the ball. Repeat 5 times on each side.

4

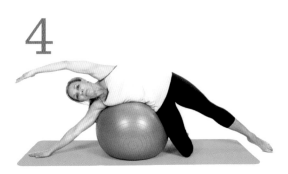

After the last repetition on each side, stretch over the ball with your arms overhead for a long side stretch. Return to starting position.

CHALLENGE YOURSELF

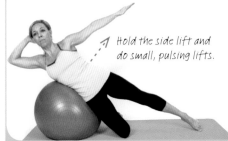

Hold the side lift and do small, pulsing lifts.

- Hold your arms overhead during side lifts for more of a challenge to your obliques and your balance.

- Hold a side lift and do small, pulsing side lifts for extra core work.

- Repeat the exercise twice on each side for additional oblique muscle strengthening.

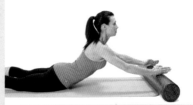

Foam Roller

This chapter contains exercises using a foam roller. For some of the exercises, the roller will help guide your motion. For others, such as helicopters, you use the foam roller to slightly lift your hips off the mat, which provides support for your body as you move your legs freely.

Both soft and firm rollers are available, and you can use either type for the exercises. If you find your foam roller to be too firm, place your mat or a towel over your roller for comfort.

mermaid

The mermaid provides a great stretch for your hips, back, and shoulders. Using the roller helps support your torso and guides your side stretch. As you do this exercise, it's important to keep your hips down on the mat to get the best stretch. Make sure you also keep your abdominals scooped during the rotation by pulling your navel away from your outer thigh; this helps you find a deeper back stretch.

BENEFITS

Improves spine flexibility
Stretches the hips and shoulders
Improves coordination

{visualize} both hips staying glued to the mat.

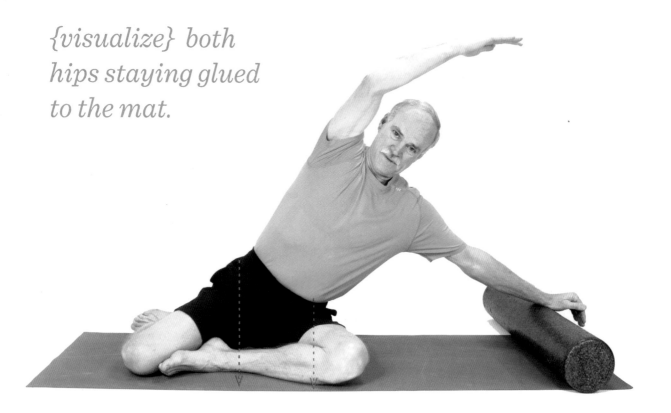

CHAPTER 14 • FOAM ROLLER

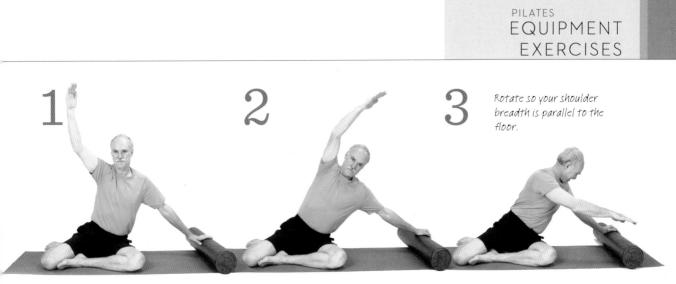

1

2

3 *Rotate so your shoulder breadth is parallel to the floor.*

Sit with one leg bent at a 90-degree angle in front of your body and your other leg bent behind you. Position the roller on the other side of the mat. Place one hand on the roller and lift your other hand straight up.

Inhale as you roll the roller away and side bend toward it.

Exhale as you rotate toward the roller, keeping your abdominals scooped. Look toward the mat and feel the stretch through your back.

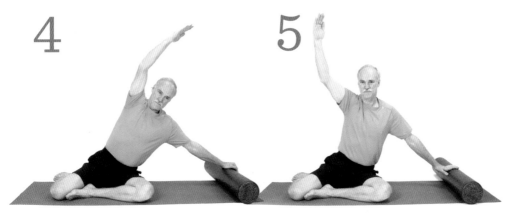

4

5

Inhale as you rotate back to the side stretch while looking straight ahead.

Exhale as you come back up to a sitting position. Repeat the exercise 5 times on each side.

MERMAID

swan with neck turns

During the swan with neck turns, the roller helps guide the movement and encourages a deeper shoulder stretch when you lower down while your arms are lifted a few inches off the mat. The swan position strengthens both your core and back, while the neck turns include a long exhale for an extra breath challenge. As you do the exercise, remember to keep your Pilates scoop throughout to protect your back.

BENEFITS

Strengthens the back and core

Stretches the shoulders

Improves spine and neck flexibility

{visualize} a string pulling your chest to the ceiling on the lift.

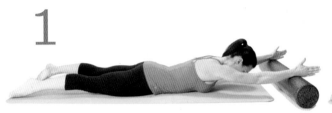

1

Lie on your stomach with your arms stretched overhead and on the foam roller, palms facing each other.

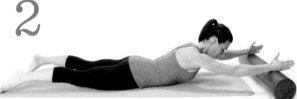

2

Draw your shoulder blades down your back as you begin an inhale, feeling the roller roll slightly toward you.

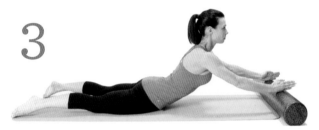

3

Continuing the inhale, arc your upper back to come to a swan position as you keep your abdominals engaged to support your lower back.

4   *Keep the roller still.*

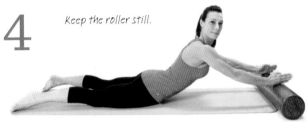

On a long exhale, look to one side.

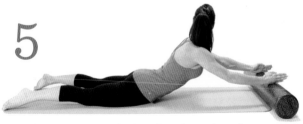

5

Continuing to exhale, look to the other side and return your head to center.

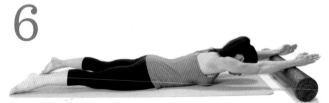

6

Lower your torso, continuing the exhale and squeezing all the air out of your lungs. The roller should stretch away from your body as you lower. Repeat the exercise 5 times.

leg scissors

Leg scissors can be done in a parallel or turnout position of the legs and work the muscles on the front and back of your legs and thighs. As you slide your legs back and forth during the exercise, brush your legs past each other and note that the two beats holding the split position is a controlled beat, not a bounce.

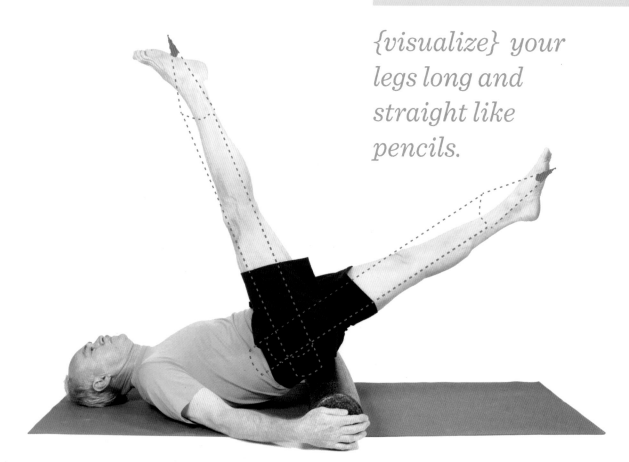

{visualize} your legs long and straight like pencils.

1

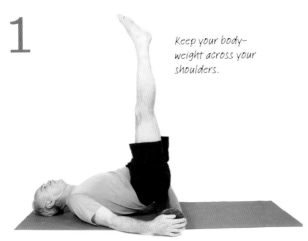

Keep your body-weight across your shoulders.

2

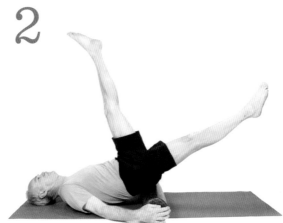

3

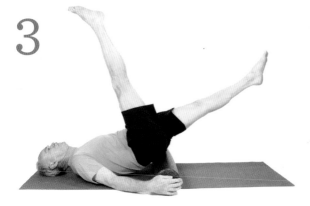

Place the foam roller under your pelvis as you engage your core muscles. Draw your legs one at a time into your chest and then extend them up to the ceiling.

Lower one leg down at a 45-degree angle while keeping your other leg up over your torso on an inhalation and hold for two small beats.

CHALLENGE YOURSELF

Press your arms into the mat with your core engaged to keep your hips lifted.

Exhale as you switch the position of your legs. Repeat the exercise 10 times before returning to starting position.

- Remove the foam roller and use your hands for support for an advanced core challenge.
- Do the exercise without the foam roller while flat on your back to strengthen your abdominals.

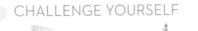

bicycles

During bicycles, you do forward and backward pedals with your legs, with one moment where both your legs are extended straight and long. As you do this exercise, be careful you never have tension going onto your neck; your bodyweight should be supported across your shoulders.

Improves lower-body flexibility

Develops lower-body coordination

Strengthens the core

{visualize} your leg pedaling a large pedal that's almost out of reach.

CHAPTER 14 • FOAM ROLLER

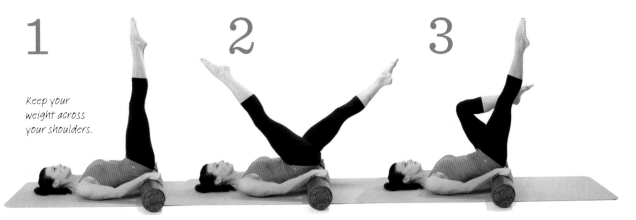

1

Keep your weight across your shoulders.

Place the foam roller under your pelvis as you engage your core muscles. Draw your legs one at a time into your chest and then extend them up to the ceiling.

2

Lower your left leg down at a 45-degree angle while your right leg comes over your torso on an inhalation.

3

Exhale as you bend and draw your left leg into your body while your right leg lowers toward the floor.

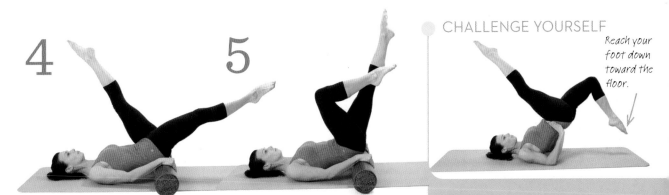

4

Inhale as you stretch both your legs long in a split position.

5

Exhale as you bend and draw your right leg into your body while your left leg lowers toward the floor. After 10 bicycles, reverse the direction of the bicycles before returning to starting position.

CHALLENGE YOURSELF

Reach your foot down toward the floor.

- Remove the foam roller and use your hands for support for an advanced core challenge.

- Lie on your back on the mat without the roller while doing this exercise to strengthen your abdominals.

BICYCLES

crisscross

During the crisscross, the roller helps support your pelvis as you work and stretch your inner thighs. Flexing your feet during the inner thigh stretch works your lower legs and allows for a deeper leg stretch. Take your time on the exhalation to squeeze all the air out of your lungs and prepare yourself for the next inhalation.

{visualize} quick crosses of your legs as you inhale.

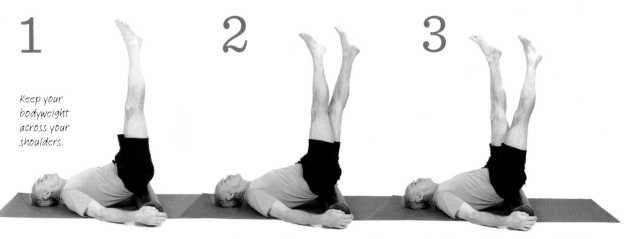

1

Keep your bodyweight across your shoulders.

Place the foam roller under your pelvis as you engage your core muscles. Draw your legs one at a time into your chest and then extend them up to the ceiling.

2

With pointed feet, cross one ankle over the other on a small inhalation.

3

Continue to inhale as you switch the cross of your legs.

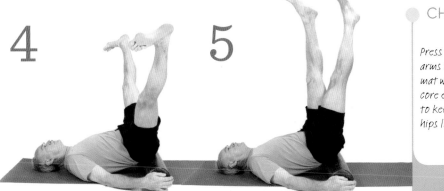

4

On a long exhale, open your legs to a wide V-stretch, flexing your feet.

5

Draw your legs back to repeat the crisscross with pointed feet. Repeat the exercise 10 times before returning to starting position.

CHALLENGE YOURSELF

Press your arms into the mat with your core engaged to keep your hips lifted.

- Remove the foam roller and use your hands for support for an advanced core challenge.

- Increase the number of crosses of your ankles, up to 10 crosses, for a deeper inhalation and extra inner-thigh work.

helicopters

Helicopters move your legs in a semicircle in opposite directions. The foam roller provides support for your pelvis and
allows for a larger helicopter motion. The circles can be kept
small to work your core or done big to work on hip flexibility.
As you do this, be sure to keep your pelvis stable and try for
a balanced position while your legs draw the circle on the
ceiling.

*{visualize} each leg drawing
reversing semicircles.*

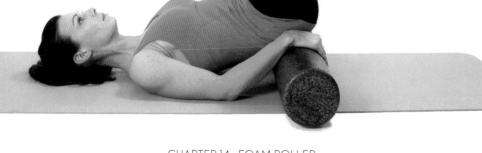

1

Keep your weight across your shoulders.

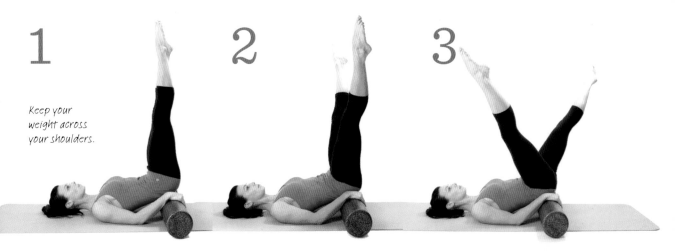

Place the foam roller under your pelvis as you engage your core muscles. Draw your legs one at a time into your chest and then extend them up to the ceiling.

2

Inhale as you stretch your legs out to a wide V-split.

3

Exhale as you move your legs in a circular motion as one of your legs goes over your torso and the other is at an angle toward the floor.

4

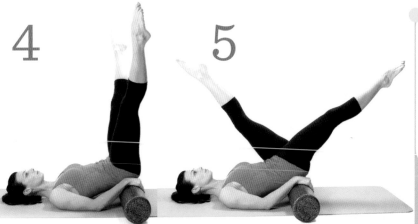

Inhale as you bring your legs back to a wide V-position, reversing the direction of the semicircle.

5

Exhale as you bring your opposite leg over your torso. Repeat the exercise 10 times before returning to starting position.

CHALLENGE YOURSELF

Press your arms into the mat.

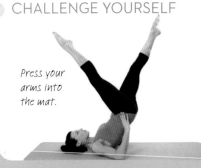

- Remove the foam roller and use your hands for support for an advanced core challenge.

- Do the exercise flat on your back on the mat to strengthen your abdominals.

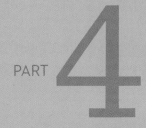

Pilates Routines

This part consists of programs that include total-body programs arranged from easiest to most challenging, sports-specific programs, and short beginner and intermediate programs that target areas of your body. All of these include exercises you learned previously in the book.

As you proceed through the programs, you will see suggested numbers of repetitions. It is more important for you to do the movement correctly than to push through an exercise in fatigue or poor form. That said, when an exercise calls for "each direction," such as "10 circles in each direction," this means you do 10 circles in a clockwise motion and then do 10 circles in a counterclockwise motion. When an exercise says "alternating sides," such as "10 times, alternating sides," this means you do 5 motions on each side of the body for a total of 10 movements.

CHAPTER 15

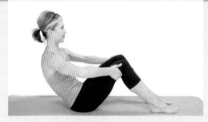

Total-Body Programs

In this chapter, you find programs that work your body from head to toe, arranged from easiest to most challenging. Each program has a suggested Pilates principle of focus. (If you recall from earlier in the book, the Pilates principles are centering, concentration, control, breath, precision, and flow of movement.) Now is your opportunity to put these principles into practice!

preparatory program

If you are looking for a simple and basic routine to start with, this preparatory program is for you. While you do the exercises, practice applying the Pilates principle of concentration, drawing your attention to how you are moving and what you are feeling in your body.

APPROXIMATE TIME

5 TO 10 MINUTES

PRINCIPLE(S) OF FOCUS

CONCENTRATION

EQUIPMENT

MAT

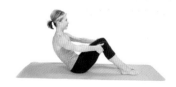

Half Rolldown
Repetitions: 10 times
Transition to next exercise:
Roll all the way down to the mat
to lie flat on your back.

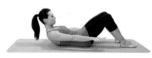

Head, Neck, and Shoulder Lift
Repetitions: 10 times
Transition to next exercise: Lower
your head so your spine is long on
the mat.

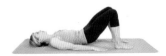

Pelvic Curl
Repetitions: 10 times
Transition to next exercise: Return to
a neutral pelvis.

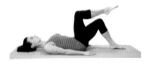

Single-Leg Lift on Your Back
Repetitions: 10 times, alternating legs
Transition to next exercise:
Roll onto your stomach.

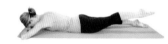

Single-Leg Lift on Your Stomach
Repetitions: 10 times, alternating legs
Transition to next exercise: Push with your arms to lift to all fours.

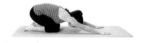

Child's Pose Stretch
Repetitions: Hold 10 to 30 seconds
Transition to next exercise:
Lift your torso and return to all fours.

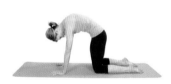

Cat
Repetitions: 5 times
Transition to next exercise:
Do a standing roll-up to come to a standing position.

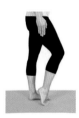

Foot Rolls and Toe Lifts
Repetitions: 10 times for each exercise
Transition to next exercise:
Stand in good alignment.

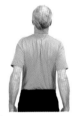

Shoulder Shrugs
Repetitions: 5 times

beginner program

In the beginner total-body program, you start by lying on your back and end in a standing position, ready for your day. Apply the Pilates principles of centering and control and continue to apply the principle of concentration, which you worked on in the preparatory program.

APPROXIMATE TIME

15 TO 20 MINUTES

PRINCIPLE(S) OF FOCUS

CENTERING AND CONTROL

EQUIPMENT

MAT

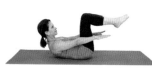

Hundred
Repetitions: 100 arm beats
Transition to next exercise: Place your feet flat and head down on the mat.

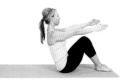

Roll-Up
Repetitions: 10 times
Transition to next exercise: End on your back on the mat.

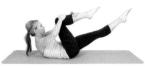

Single-Leg Stretch
Repetitions: 10 times, alternating legs
Transition to next exercise: Finish with both your knees to your chest.

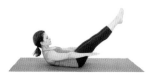

Double-Leg Stretch
Repetitions: 10 times
Transition to next exercise: Place your feet on the mat with your knees bent and your feet close to your pelvis.

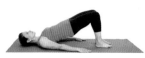

Double-Leg Bridge
Repetitions: 10 times
Transition to next exercise: Finish on your back with your knees bent.

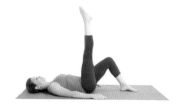

Leg Circles
Repetitions: 10 times in each direction
Transition to next exercise: Roll onto your side.

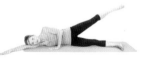

Leg Lift and Lower
Repetitions: 10 times
Transition to next exercise: Do the front and back sweeps before turning over to do both exercises on the other side.

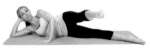

Front and Back Sweeps
Repetitions: 10 times
Transition to next exercise: Roll onto your stomach.

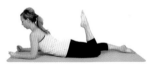

Single-Leg Kick
Repetitions: 10 times, alternating legs
Transition to next exercise: Lower your upper body to the mat and place your hands on the mat, just above your shoulders.

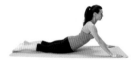

Swan
Repetitions: 5 times
Transition to next exercise: Do a child's pose stretch, if desired, and come up on all fours.

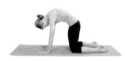

Cat
Repetitions: 5 times
Transition to next exercise: Remain in the all-fours position.

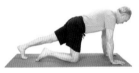

All Fours to Plank
Repetitions: 5 times
Transition to next exercise: Come to a seated position at the front of your mat and bring your knees to your chest.

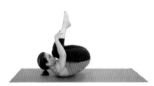

Rolling Like a Ball
Repetitions: 10 times
Transition to next exercise: Finish in a seated position and place your feet on the mat in a V-position.

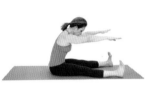

Spine Stretch
Repetitions: 10 times
Transition to next exercise: Bend your legs into a diamond and press the bottoms of your feet together.

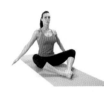

Circles in the Sand
Repetitions: 10 times, alternating sides

intermediate program

This program builds on the exercises from the beginner program, so be sure you are proficient with the beginner program first. During the challenging core and upper-body exercises, try to incorporate the Pilates principles of breath and precision—work on connecting your breath to your movement, and try to perform the exercises as precisely as possible.

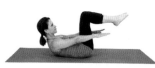

Hundred
Repetitions: 100 arm beats
Transition to next exercise: Lower your head and place your feet flat on the mat with your knees bent.

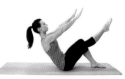

Teaser Prep
Repetitions: 5 times
Transition to next exercise: Bend your knees to your chest and lift your head, neck, and shoulders.

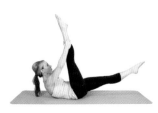

Straight-Leg Pull
Repetitions: 10 times, alternating legs
Transition to next exercise: Return your knees back to your chest and place your hands behind your head.

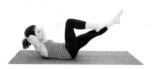

Crisscross
Repetitions: 10 times, alternating sides
Transition to next exercise: Lift your legs to a 90-degree angle at your hip with your arms at the sides of your body and lifted off the mat.

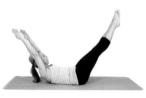

Double-Leg Lifts
Repetitions: 10 times
Transition to next exercise: Roll up to come to a sitting position.

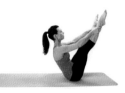

Open-Leg Rocker
Repetitions: 10 times
Transition to next exercise: Roll down to the mat to lie flat on your back, knees bent and feet flat on the floor.

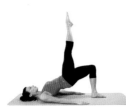

Single-Leg Bridge Kicks
Repetitions: 10 times, alternating legs
Transition to next exercise:
Straighten your legs on the mat.

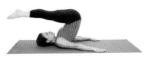

Rollover
Repetitions: 5 times
Transition to next exercise:
Roll onto your side.

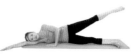

Side-Lying Leg Circles
Repetitions: 10 times in each direction
Transition to next exercise: Remain on
your side.

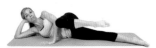

Side-Lying Bicycles
Repetitions: 10 times
Transition to next exercise:
Remain on your side and bring your
top leg to a turnout position.

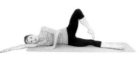

Side-Lying Leg Develope
Repetitions: 10 times
Transition to next exercise: Remain
on your side and bend your top leg in
front of your bottom thigh with your
foot flat on the mat.

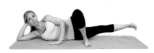

Inner Thigh Lifts
Repetitions: 10 times
Transition to next exercise: Repeat the
three previous side-lying exercises
and this exercise on your other side.
Roll onto your stomach when you're
done.

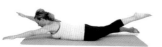

Swimming

Repetitions: 50 times, alternating beats, or 5 cycles of breathing
Transition to next exercise: Place your hands on the small of your back and turn your head, resting on the mat, to one side.

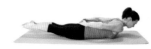

Double-Leg Kick

Repetitions: 10 times, alternating sides
Transition to next exercise: Do a child's pose stretch, if desired, and come up on all fours.

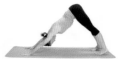

Plank to V-Stretch

Repetitions: 10 times
Transition to next exercise: Sit on the mat with your legs open in a small V-position.

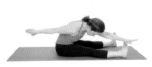

Saw

Repetitions: 10 times, alternating sides
Transition to next exercise: While sitting, place your hands behind you and bring your knees to your chest.

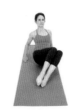

Can-Can

Repetitions: 10 times, alternating sides
Transition to next exercise: Bring your legs in a bent position to the side and stretch over your legs.

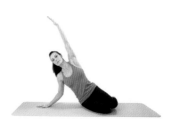

Mermaid

Repetitions: 5 times on each side
Transition to next exercise: Bring your legs to a small V-position on the mat and grab your arm weights, if desired.

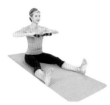

Rowing 1
Repetitions: 10 times
Transition to next exercise: Bring your arms down to the sides of your body, palms up and elbows bent.

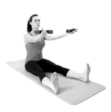

Serve a Tray
Repetitions: 10 times
Transition to next exercise: Do a standing roll-up to come to a standing position.

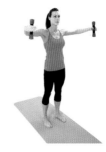

Hug a Tree
Repetitions: 10 times for each breath pattern
Transition to next exercise: Remain in a standing position and set your arm weights to the side.

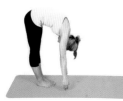

Standing Rolldown
Repetitions: 5 times
Transition to next exercise: Return to standing and roll to the ball of one foot.

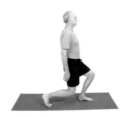

Single-Knee Bends
Repetitions: 10 times on each side

advanced program

Before attempting the advanced program, make sure you have a strong core by mastering the beginner and intermediate programs. While you do this program, incorporate the Pilates principle of flow of movement, moving from one exercise to the next with grace. If you find any of the exercises in this program too difficult, feel free to pick a substitute exercise from an earlier program.

APPROXIMATE TIME

30 TO 40 MINUTES

PRINCIPLE(S) OF FOCUS

FLOW OF MOVEMENT

EQUIPMENT

MAT AND FOAM ROLLER

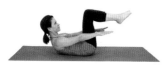

Hundred
Repetitions: 100 arm beats
Transition to next exercise: Straighten your legs flat on the mat.

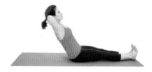

Neck Pull
Repetitions: 5 times
Transition to next exercise: Roll down to the mat and pull your knees to your chest.

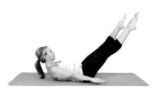

Coordination
Repetitions: 10 times
Transition to next exercise: Extend your legs out to a 45-degree angle.

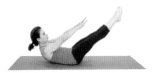

Teaser 1
Repetitions: 5 times
Transition to next exercise: Lower your torso and legs to the mat.

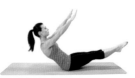

Teaser 2
Repetitions: 5 times
Transition to next exercise: Roll up to a sitting position.

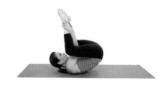

Seal
Repetitions: 10 times
Transition to next exercise: Move onto your stomach and place your hands on the mat just above your shoulders.

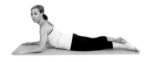

Swan with Neck Rolls
Repetitions: Neck rolls 5 times in each
direction
Transition to next exercise: Rest your
head on your hands.

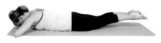

Heel Beats
Repetitions: 50 beats or 5 cycles of
breathing
Transition to next exercise: Bend your
knees and lift your torso.

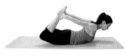

Rocker Position
Repetitions: Hold for 5 cycles of
breathing
Transition to next exercise: If desired,
do the child's pose stretch and a
standing roll-up to come to a standing
position.

Push-Up
Repetitions: 5 times
Transition to next exercise: Hold a
plank position.

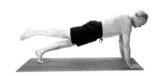

Leg Pull Front
Repetitions: 10 leg lifts, alternating legs
Transition to next exercise: Turn over
and sit on the mat with your hands
behind you.

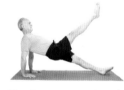

Leg Pullback
Repetitions: 10 leg lifts, alternating legs
Transition to next exercise: Roll down to
the mat.

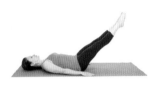

Corkscrew
Repetitions: 10 times in each direction
Transition to next exercise: Lower
your legs to the mat.

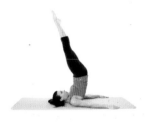

Jackknife
Repetitions: 5 times
Transition to next exercise: Do a roll-
up to come to a sitting position.

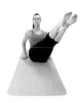

Modified Hip Circles
Repetitions: 5 times in each direction
Transition to next exercise: Sit with
your legs straight in front of you on
the mat.

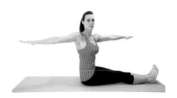

Spine Twist
Repetitions: 10 times, alternating sides
Transition to next exercise: Bring one
leg in front of your torso and bend
your other leg to the side to come to a
fourth position.

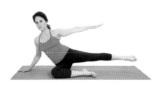

Seated Fourth Glute Work
Repetitions: 10 times on each side
Transition to next exercise: Come to a
kneeling position.

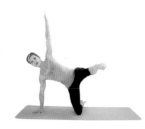

Kneeling Side Kicks
Repetitions: 10 times on each side
Transition to next exercise: Place your
feet to the side with your top leg to
the back.

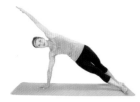

Side Bend
Repetitions: 5 times
Transition to next exercise: From a
side plank position, move straight into
the next exercise.

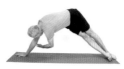

Twist
Repetitions: 5 times
Transition to next exercise: Turn over
and repeat the side bend and this exercise on your other side. Move onto
your back with the foam roller under
your hips.

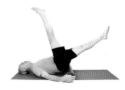

Leg Scissors
Repetitions: 10 times, alternating sides
Transition to next exercise: Remain on
the foam roller.

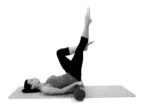

Bicycles
Repetitions: 10 times in each direction
Transition to next exercise: Bring your
legs straight up to the ceiling.

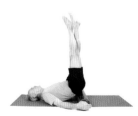

Crisscross
Repetitions: 10 times
Transition to next exercise: Hold your
legs in a wide V-position.

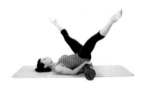

Helicopters
Repetitions: 10 times
Transition to next exercise: Slowly
push the roller out from under your
hips to lie flat on the mat. Bring both
your legs up to the ceiling.

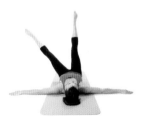

Single-Side Leg Lower and Lift
Repetitions: 10 times, alternating sides
Transition to next exercise: Keep your
legs up to the ceiling with a 90-degree
angle at your hips.

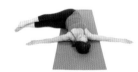

Double-Side Leg Lower and Lift
Repetitions: 10 times, alternating
sides

CHAPTER 16

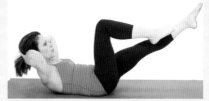

Sports Programs

The programs in this chapter focus on target areas needed for a specific sport—running, swimming, cycling, golf, or tennis. All of these short sports programs include core strengthening and work on flexibility (for more-extensive programs, check out the previous total-body programs). Each of the programs starts with the hundred, which is a perfect opportunity to put your breath work to practice! Throughout the programs, remember to breathe deeply through your nose and exhale out your mouth.

running program

This running program focuses on your core strength and lower body, starting on the mat with abdominal work and ending with standing footwork. Because your feet act as your base of support, pay attention to the alignment of your body and legs. Keeping a strong core and staying in good alignment can help take the stress off your joints as you run.

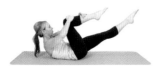

Hundred
Repetitions: 100 arm beats
Transition to next exercise: Place your feet flat, knees bent, and your head, neck, and shoulders down on the mat.

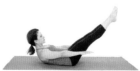

Roll-Up
Repetitions: 10 times
Transition to next exercise: Roll down to the mat to lie flat on your back.

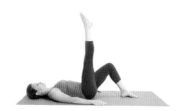

Leg Circles
Repetitions: 10 times in each direction
Transition to next exercise: Lift your head, neck, and shoulders and pull your knees to your chest.

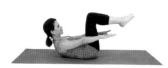

Single-Leg Stretch
Repetitions: 10 times, alternating legs
Transition to next exercise: Draw both your knees to your chest.

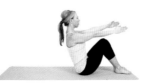

Double-Leg Stretch
Repetitions: 10 times
Transition to next exercise: Roll onto your side.

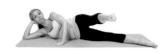

Front and Back Sweeps
Repetitions: 10 times
Transition to next exercise: Stay on your side.

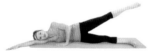

Side-Lying Leg Circles

Repetitions: 10 times in each direction
Transition to next exercise: Remain on
your side.

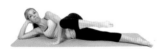

Side-Lying Bicycles

Repetitions: 10 times
Transition to next exercise: Stay on
the same side and bend your top leg,
foot flat on the mat and in front of
your thigh.

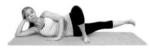

Inner Thigh Lifts

Repetitions: 10 times
Transition to next exercise: Repeat
the previous exercises, from front and
back sweeps to this exercise, on your
other side. Roll onto your stomach.

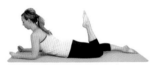

Single-Leg Kick

Repetitions: 10 times, alternating legs
Transition to next exercise: Come up
on all fours.

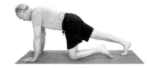

All Fours to Plank

Repetitions: 5 times
Transition to next exercise: Hold a
plank position.

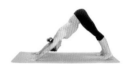

Plank to V-Stretch

Repetitions: 10 times
Transition to next exercise: Return to
all fours using all fours to plank and
lower to a side-sit position on the mat.

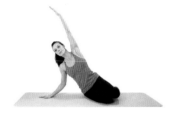

Mermaid

Repetitions: 5 times on each side
Transition to next exercise: Come to a
standing position.

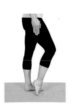

Foot Rolls and Toe Lifts

Repetitions: 10 times for each exercise

swimming program

This swimming program includes several exercises that allow you to work on your breath control, such as the hundred, swimming, and heel beats. You are welcome to increase the number of breath parts from 5 parts to 6 or more parts to challenge your breath control and lung capacity even more.

APPROXIMATE TIME

15 TO 20 MINUTES

AREAS OF FOCUS

CORE STRENGTH, BREATH CONTROL, AND UPPER-BODY FLEXIBILITY AND STRENGTH

EQUIPMENT

MAT, SMALL ARM WEIGHTS (IF DESIRED), AND BAND/POLE

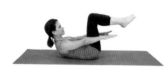

Hundred
Repetitions: 100 arm beats
Transition to next exercise: Place your feet flat, knees bent, and your head, neck, and shoulders down on the mat.

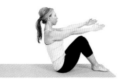

Roll-Up
Repetitions: 10 times
Transition to next exercise: Roll down to the mat to lie flat on your back.

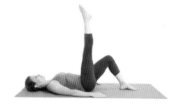

Leg Circles
Repetitions: 10 times in each direction
Transition to next exercise: Lift your head, neck, and shoulders and pull your knees to your chest.

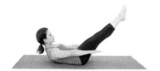

Double-Leg Stretch
Repetitions: 10 times
Transition to next exercise: Lower your head and place your feet on the mat, knees bent.

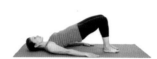

Double-Leg Bridge
Repetitions: 10 times
Transition to next exercise: Do a roll-up to come up to a sitting position. Hold arm weights in your hands, if desired.

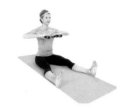

Rowing 1
Repetitions: 10 times
Transition to next exercise: Continue sitting.

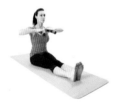

Rowing 2
Repetitions: 10 times
Transition to next exercise: Continue sitting and hinge forward slightly at your hips, keeping your spine straight.

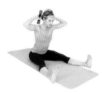

Shaving
Repetitions: 10 times
Transition to next exercise: Come on all fours with an arm weight in one of your hands, if desired.

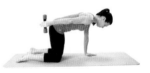

Pullbacks and Tricep Extensions
Repetitions: 10 times
Transition to next exercise: Lower to the mat to lie on your stomach.

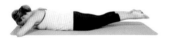

Heel Beats
Repetitions: 5 cycles of breathing or 50 beats
Transition to next exercise: Stay on your stomach and bring your arms overhead.

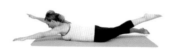

Swimming
Repetitions: 5 cycles of breathing
Transition to next exercise: Do a child's pose stretch, if desired. Do a standing roll-up to come to a standing position with a band or pole in your hands.

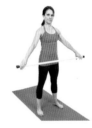

Front Arm Lifts
Repetitions: 10 times
Transition to next exercise: Hold a band or pole overhead.

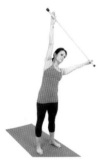

Side Stretch
Repetitions: 10 times, alternating sides
Transition to next exercise: Continue to hold the band or pole over your head.

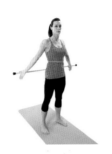

Behind-the-Back Arm Bends
Repetitions: 10 times

biking program

In this program, you work on both your upper and lower body, in addition to your core strength, to prepare and strengthen your biking. Because your body position when biking has your hips bent and your arms forward, this program also works on opening your chest and stretching the front of your hips to encourage good posture.

APPROXIMATE TIME

15 TO 20 MINUTES

AREAS OF FOCUS

CORE STRENGTH, FLEXIBILITY, LOWER-BODY STRENGTH, AND UPPER-BODY STABILITY

EQUIPMENT

MAT, SMALL ARM WEIGHTS (IF DESIRED), AND BAND/POLE

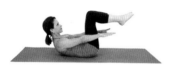

Hundred
Repetitions: 100 arm beats
Transition to next exercise: Place your feet flat, knees bent, and your head, neck, and shoulders down on the mat.

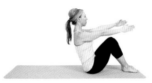

Roll-Up
Repetitions: 10 times
Transition to next exercise: Roll down to the mat to lie flat on your back.

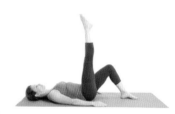

Leg Circles
Repetitions: 10 times in each direction
Transition to next exercise: Lift your head, neck, and shoulders and pull your knees to your chest.

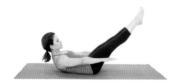

Double-Leg Stretch
Repetitions: 10 times
Transition to next exercise: With both legs straight, extend one of your legs to the ceiling and your other leg at a low angle.

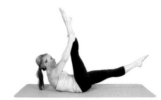

Straight-Leg Pull
Repetitions: 10 times, alternating legs
Transition to next exercise: Roll onto your side.

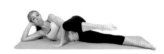

Side-Lying Bicycles
Repetitions: 10 times
Transition to next exercise: Stay on the same side and turn out your top leg.

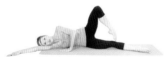

Side-Lying Leg Develope
Repetitions: 10 times
Transition to next exercise: Bend your top leg up and place your foot flat on the floor in front of your thigh.

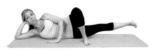

Inner Thigh Lifts
Repetitions: 10 times
Transition to next exercise: Repeat the previous exercises, from side-lying bicycles to this exercise, on your other side. Roll onto your stomach.

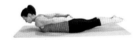

Double-Leg Kick
Repetitions: 10 times, alternating sides
Transition to next exercise: Stay on your stomach and place your hands on the mat.

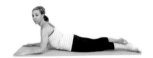

Swan with Neck Rolls
Repetitions: 5 neck rolls each way
Transition to next exercise: Stay on your stomach while bending your knees and reaching back for your ankles.

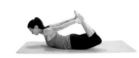

Rocker Position
Repetitions: Hold for 5 cycles of breathing
Transition to next exercise: Come on all fours and do a child's pose stretch, if desired.

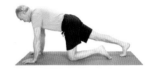

All Fours to Plank
Repetitions: 5 times
Transition to next exercise: Hold a plank position.

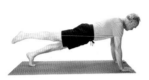

Leg Pull Front
Repetitions: 10 leg lifts, alternating legs
Transition to next exercise: Return to all fours and do a standing roll-up to come to a standing position.

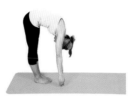

Standing Rolldown
Repetitions: 5 times

golf program

During this golf program, you use a large ball to develop control and balance, which should help you with the accuracy needed during some of your shorter shots. This program also includes exercises that work on the flexibility of your hips, spine, and shoulders for good swing mechanics and more driving distance off the tee..

APPROXIMATE TIME

15 TO 20 MINUTES

AREAS OF FOCUS

CORE STRENGTH, FLEXIBILITY, BALANCE, ROTATION, AND HIP STRENGTH AND CONTROL

EQUIPMENT

MAT, LARGE BALL, AND RING

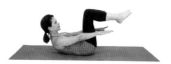

Hundred
Repetitions: 100 arm beats
Transition to next exercise: Pull your knees to your chest and lift your head, neck, and shoulders. Extend one of your legs out at a 45-degree angle.

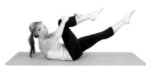

Single-Leg Stretch
Repetitions: 10 times, alternating legs
Transition to next exercise: Bend both knees to your chest.

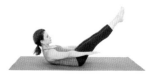

Double-Leg Stretch
Repetitions: 10 times
Transition to next exercise: Bring your hands behind your head and extend one of your legs out to a 45-degree angle.

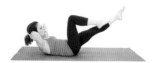

Crisscross
Repetitions: 10 times, alternating sides
Transition to next exercise: Do a standing roll-up to come to a standing position. Hold the ring in your hands.

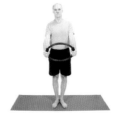

Press and Pull
Repetitions: 10 times in each position
Transition to next exercise: Set aside the ring. Come to a bridge position with your neck and shoulders supported by the ball.

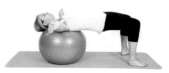

Bridge with Arm Circles
Repetitions: 5 circles in each direction
Transition to next exercise: Sit on the ball.

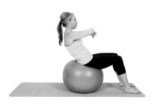

Round Back and Round Back with Twist

Repetitions: 10 times for each exercise
Transition to next exercise: Kneel next to the ball, keeping the ball to your side.

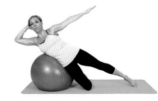

Side Lifts

Repetitions: 5 times on each side
Transition to next exercise: Come to a plank position with the ball under the front of your legs.

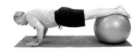

Plank Push-Ups and Shoulder Slides

Repetitions: 10 times for each exercise
Transition to next exercise: Lie on the mat with the back of your legs on the ball.

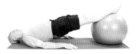

Bridges with Feet on Ball

Repetitions: 10 times
Transition to next exercise: Put aside the ball. Roll up to a sitting position and draw your legs together on the mat.

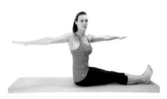

Spine Twist

Repetitions: 10 times, alternating sides
Transition to next exercise: Continue sitting and bring your legs to a small V-position. Place the ring upright in front of your body.

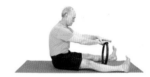

Spine Stretch

Repetitions: 10 times
Transition to next exercise: Lie on your stomach with the ring between your ankles.

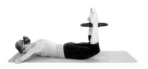

Butt Blasters

Repetitions: 10 times
Transition to next exercise: Do a child's pose stretch, if desired, and roll onto your back. Bring your legs up to the ceiling at a 90-degree angle to your hips.

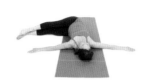

Double-Side Leg Lower and Lift

Repetitions: 10 times, alternating sides

tennis program

This is one of the more-challenging sports programs in this chapter. The tennis program works on the core strength and flexibility needed to hit a tennis ball from any angle. As there are many quick changes in direction and an immense variety of swing angles, a strong core is necessary to make these changes. Your serve, forehand, and backhand will thank you for the extra flexibility and strength.

APPROXIMATE TIME

15 TO 20 MINUTES

AREAS OF FOCUS

CORE STRENGTH, FLEXIBILITY, ROTATION, AND UPPER- AND LOWER-BODY STRENGTH

EQUIPMENT

MAT

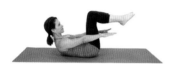

Hundred
Repetitions: 100 arm beats
Transition to next exercise: Place your feet flat, knees bent, and your head, neck, and shoulders down on the mat.

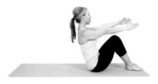

Roll-Up
Repetitions: 10 times
Transition to next exercise: Roll down to the mat to lie flat on your back. Lift your head, neck, and shoulders and pull your knees to your chest. Extend one leg at a 45-degree angle.

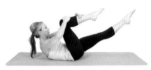

Single-Leg Stretch
Repetitions: 10 times, alternating legs
Transition to next exercise: Bring your hands behind your head.

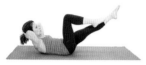

Crisscross
Repetitions: 10 times, alternating sides
Transition to next exercise: Lower your head to the mat and extend your legs at a 90-degree angle to your hip.

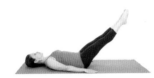

Corkscrew
Repetitions: 10 circles in each direction
Transition to next exercise: Roll up to a sitting position and bend your knees to your chest with a rounded spine.

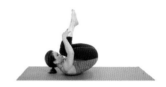

Rolling Like a Ball
Repetitions: 10 times
Transition to next exercise: Lower your legs to the mat in a small V-position.

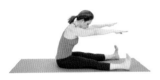

Spine Stretch
Repetitions: 10 times
Transition to next exercise: Continue sitting with your legs in a small V-position.

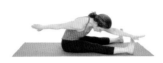

Saw
Repetitions: 10 times, alternating sides
Transition to next exercise: Stay seated with your hands behind you on the mat. Bend your knees to your chest with your toes touching the mat.

Can-Can
Repetitions: 10 times, alternating sides
Transition to next exercise: Stay seated with your arms behind you and your knees bent with your toes touching the mat.

Modified Hip Circles
Repetitions: 5 times in each direction
Transition to next exercise: Keep your arms behind you and straighten your legs on the mat.

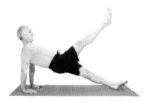

Leg Pullback
Repetitions: 10 alternating leg lifts
Transition to next exercise: Turn over to come on all fours and do all fours to plank to come to a front plank.

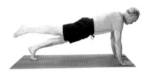

Leg Pull Front
Repetitions: 10 alternating leg lifts
Transition to next exercise: Lower yourself to the mat to lie on your stomach.

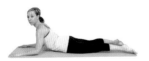

Swan with Neck Rolls
Repetitions: 5 neck rolls in each direction
Transition to next exercise: Push up with your arms.

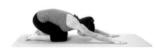

Child's Pose Stretch
Repetitions: Hold 10 to 30 seconds

CHAPTER 17

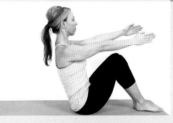

To the Point: Short Routines

The programs in this chapter are great for some quick work to a certain body area. This chapter contains four focuses: abdominals, lower body, upper body, and flexibility. Even though the focus of the work is on one area for each, keep in mind that Pilates exercises should challenge your entire body. Therefore, be attentive to the alignment of the rest of your body. There are beginner and intermediate programs for each targeted area, so start with the beginner programs before moving to the more-challenging programs.

abdominals

These programs work all of your abdominal muscles: *transverse abdominis* (a significant part of what makes up your core), *rectus abdominis* (also known as your "six-pack muscles") and internal and external obliques (found on each side of your stomach). If your abdominals fatigue during these exercises, you may start feeling the work in your back. If you feel any of these exercises in your back, stop and rest.

APPROXIMATE TIME

5 TO 8 MINUTES (BEGINNER)
8 TO 12 MINUTES (INTERMEDIATE)

TARGET AREA

ABDOMINALS

EQUIPMENT

MAT

beginner

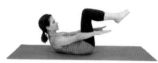

Hundred
Repetitions: 100 arm beats
Transition to next exercise: Lower your head and place your feet on the mat.

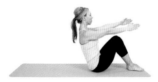

Roll-Up
Repetitions: 10 times
Transition to next exercise: Roll down to the mat and draw your knees to your chest.

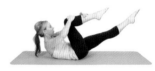

Single-Leg Stretch
Repetitions: 10 times, alternating legs
Transition to next exercise: Draw both your knees to your chest and keep your head, neck, and shoulders lifted.

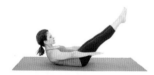

Double-Leg Stretch
Repetitions: 10 times
Transition to next exercise: Bring your hands behind your head and extend one leg long at a 45-degree angle.

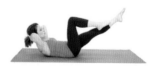

Crisscross
Repetitions: 10 times, alternating sides
Transition to next exercise: Do a roll-up to come to a sitting position.

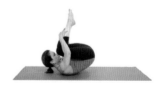

Rolling Like a Ball
Repetitions: 10 times

intermediate

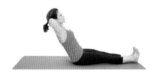

Neck Pull
Repetitions: 5 times
Transition to next exercise: Lower
your torso to the mat and extend one
of your legs at a 45-degree angle as
your other leg comes over your torso.

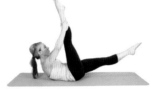

Straight-Leg Pull
Repetitions: 10 times, alternating legs
Transition to next exercise: Bring your
legs up to the ceiling at a 90-degree
angle with your hip. Extend your arms
long off the mat with your hands at
the sides of your hips.

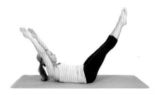

Double-Leg Lifts
Repetitions: 10 times
Transition to next exercise: Lower
your head and your legs to lie long on
your back on the mat.

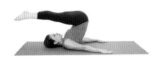

Rollover
Repetitions: 5 times
Transition to next exercise: Bring your
legs up to the ceiling at a 90-degree
angle with your hips flat on the mat
and your arms resting by your sides.

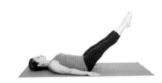

Corkscrew
Repetitions: 10 times in each direction
Transition to next exercise: Do a roll-
up to come to a sitting position.

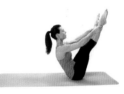

Open-Leg Rocker
Repetitions: 10 times
Transition to next exercise: Bend your
knees, keeping the tips of your toes on
the mat. Support your torso with your
hands behind you.

Modified Hip Circles
Repetitions: 5 times in each direction
Transition to next exercise: Get on
your stomach.

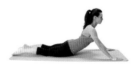

Swan
Repetitions: 5 times

lower body

Both programs work the muscles of your feet, glutes, and inner thighs. They start in a standing position and then move to exercises on your back on the mat. During the exercises, remember to keep your Pilates scoop for core stability and strengthening. When transitioning from standing to lying on your back, use the standing rolldown and the roll-up.

APPROXIMATE TIME

5 TO 8 MINUTES (BEGINNER);
8 TO 12 MINUTES (INTERMEDIATE)

TARGET AREA

LOWER BODY

EQUIPMENT

MAT (BEGINNER); MAT, FOAM
ROLLER, AND RING (INTERMEDIATE)

beginner

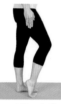

Foot Rolls and Toe Lifts
Repetitions: 10 times for each exercise
Transition to next exercise: Come from a standing position to lie flat on your back.

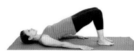

Double-Leg Bridge
Repetitions: 10 times
Transition to next exercise: Come to a side-lying position.

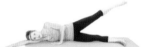

Leg Lift and Lower
Repetitions: 10 times
Transition to next exercise: Continue lying on the same side.

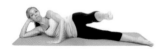

Front and Back Sweeps
Repetitions: 10 times
Transition to next exercise: Continue lying on the same side.

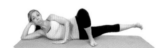

Inner Thigh Lifts
Repetitions: 10 times
Transition to next exercise: Roll onto your other side and repeat from leg lift and lower to here. When done, roll onto your stomach, supporting your torso with your elbows.

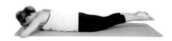

Heel Beats
Repetitions: 50 beats or 5 cycles of breathing

intermediate

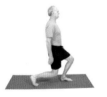

Single-Knee Bends
Repetitions: 10 on each side
Transition to next exercise: Come
from a standing position to lie flat on
your back.

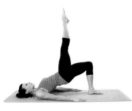

Single-Leg Bridge Kicks
Repetitions: 10 times, alternating sides
Transition to next exercise: Come to
a bridge position and place the roller
under your pelvis.

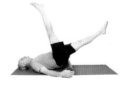

Leg Scissors
Repetitions: 10 times, alternating legs
Transition to next exercise: Hold a leg
scissor and bend the leg farthest from
your body to begin.

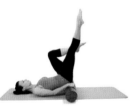

Bicycles
Repetitions: 10 times in each direction
Transition to next exercise: Bring your
legs straight up to the ceiling.

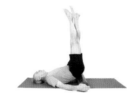

Crisscross
Repetitions: 10 times
Transition to next exercise: Hold your
legs in a wide V-position.

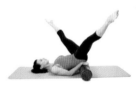

Helicopters
Repetitions: 10 times
Transition to next exercise: Come to
a side-lying position with your bottom
leg inside the ring.

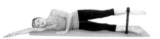

Inner Thigh Presses and Glute Pulls
Repetitions: 10 times on each side for each exercise
Transition to next exercise: Roll onto your stomach with the
ring between your ankles.

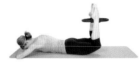

Butt Blasters
Repetitions: 10 times

upper body

Both the beginner and intermediate programs can be done with or without arm weights and are a great workout for the front and back of your arms, shoulders, midback, and core. The beginner upper-body program will use weights, if desired, and a band or pole. The intermediate program will not only use arm weights but also your bodyweight for resistance during planks, which will strengthen your core.

beginner

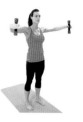

Hug a Tree
Repetitions: 10 times for each breath pattern
Transition to next exercise: Continue standing with arm weights in your hands and your arms resting at your sides.

Arm Circles
Repetitions: 10 times in each direction
Transition to next exercise: Do a standing rolldown to sit on the mat. Bring your arms to the sides of your ribcage, palms up.

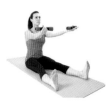

Serve a Tray
Repetitions: 10 times
Transition to next exercise: Come on all fours with an arm weight in one of your hands.

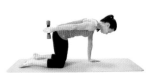

Pullbacks and Tricep Extensions
Repetitions: 10 times on each side for each exercise
Transition to next exercise: After each arm, do a standing roll-up and hold onto a band or pole.

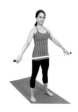

Front Arm Lifts
Repetitions: 10 times
Transition to next exercise: Hold the band or pole overhead.

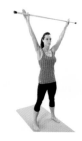

Overhead Arm Press
Repetitions: 10 times

intermediate

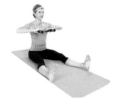

Rowing 1
Repetitions: 10 times
Transition to next exercise: Sit on the mat with your legs together.

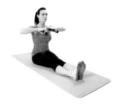

Rowing 2
Repetitions: 10 times
Transition to next exercise: Do all fours to plank to come to a plank position.

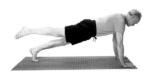

Leg Pull Front
Repetitions: 10 alternating leg lifts
Transition to next exercise: Turn over with your hands behind you on the mat.

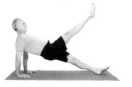

Leg Pullback
Repetitions: 10 alternating leg lifts
Transition to next exercise: Come onto your side with your feet, hips, shoulders, and hands in a straight line.

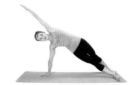

Side Bend
Repetitions: 5 times on each side
Transition to next exercise: Come to a plank with your legs on the ball.

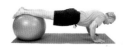

Plank Push-Ups and Shoulder Slides
Repetitions: 10 times for each exercise
Transition to next exercise: Lie on the ball with your upper back and head supported by it.

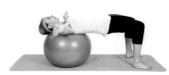

Bridge with Arm Circles
Repetitions: 5 times in each direction

flexibility

Many Pilates exercises stretch and strengthen your muscles simultaneously through fluid movement. While you are using the Pilates exercises with a flexibility focus in both the beginner and intermediate programs, feel free to hold positions for a stretch of 10 to 30 seconds. Holding a stretch gives your tissues and muscles extra time to lengthen, improving your flexibility more quickly.

beginner

Circles in the Sand
Repetitions: 10 times, alternating sides
Transition to next exercise: Open your legs to a V-position while still sitting on the mat.

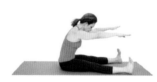

Spine Stretch
Repetitions: 10 times
Transition to next exercise: Roll down to the mat and bring both your legs up to the ceiling at a 90-degree angle to your hips.

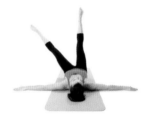

Single-Side Leg Lower and Lift
Repetitions: 10 times, alternating sides
Transition to next exercise: Come onto all fours.

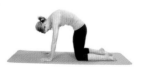

Cat
Repetitions: 5 times
Transition to next exercise: Lower to the mat on your stomach.

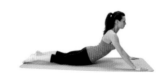

Swan
Repetitions: 5 times
Transition to next exercise: Push up with your hands to bring your hips toward your heels.

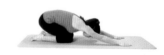

Child's Pose Stretch
Repetitions: Hold 10 to 30 seconds

intermediate

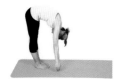

Standing Rolldown
Repetitions: 5 times
Transition to next exercise: Hold a
rolldown to bend your knees and sit
on the mat. Come to a fourth position
with a foam roller to the side of your
body.

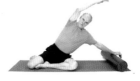

Mermaid
Repetitions: 5 times each way
Transition to next exercise: Get onto
your stomach with your arms on the
foam roller overhead.

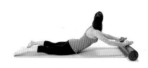

Swan with Neck Turns
Repetitions: 5 times
Transition to next exercise: Reach
your arms back toward your ankles as
you bend your knees.

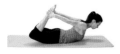

Rocker Position
Repetitions: Hold for 5 cycles of
breathing
Transition to next exercise: Come to a
plank position.

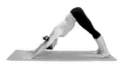

Plank to V-Stretch
Repetitions: 10 times
Transition to next exercise: Sit on the
mat with your legs in a V-position.

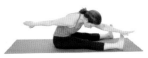

Saw
Repetitions: 10 times, alternating sides
Transition to next exercise: Roll down
to the mat to lie on your back.

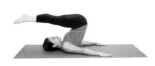

Rollover
Repetitions: 5 times
Transition to next exercise: Remain on your back and bring
your legs to a 90-degree angle at your hip.

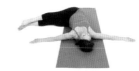

Double-Side Leg Lower and Lift
Repetitions: 10 times, alternating sides

index

A

abdominals
    ab work with ring in hands, 180–181
    all fours to plank, 136–137
    bridges with feet on ball, 216–217
    can-can, 110–111
    cat, 138–139
    circles in the sand, 116–117
    coordination, 56–57
    corkscrew, 54–55
    crisscross, 50–51
    double-leg stretch, 46–47
    hundred, 38–39
    jackknife, 60–61
    leg pullback, 144–145
    modified hip circles, 112–113
    neck pull, 62–63
    Pilates scoop, 26
    plank to v-stretch, 150–151
    push-up, 142–143
    rollover, 58–59
    roll-up, 40–41
    round back/round back with twist (fitness ball), 218–219
    short routine, 268–269
    single-leg stretch, 44–45
    spine stretch (ring), 172–173
    spine twist, 104–105
    straight-leg pull, 48–49
    teaser 1, 66–67
    teaser 2, 68–69
    teaser prep, 64–65
    transverse abdominis, 26
adaptations, 9
advanced program, 250–253
alignment, 11–23
all-fours position, 135–139
all fours to plank, 136–137
arm weights, 164, 183–197
    arm circles, 190–191
    hug a tree, 184–185
    pullbacks, 196–197
    rowing 1, 186–187
    rowing 2, 188–189
    serve a tray, 192–193
    shaving, 194–195
    tricep extension, 196–197
arms
    alignment, 20–21
    arm circles (weights), 190–191
    jackknife, 60–61
    plank push-ups (fitness ball), 220–221
    pullbacks (weights), 196–197
    serve a tray (weights), 192–193
    shaving (weights), 194–195
    shoulder slides (fitness ball), 220–221
    tricep extension (weights), 196–197

B

back
    cat, 138–139
    circles in the sand, 116–117
    double-leg kick, 122–123
    mat work, 37–83
    plank push-ups (fitness ball), 220–221
    rocker position, 130–131
    shoulder slides (fitness ball), 220–221
    side stretch (band/pole), 208–209
    swan, 126–127
    swan with neck rolls, 128–129
    swan with neck turns (foam roller), 228–229
    swimming, 124–125
balance
    bridge with arm circles (fitness ball), 214–215
    foot rolls and toe lifts, 158–159
    kneeling side kicks, 98–99
    modified hip circles, 112–113
    open-leg rocker, 76–77
    plank push-ups (fitness ball), 220–221
    rolling like a ball, 74–75
    round back/round back with twist (fitness ball), 218–219
    seal, 78–79
    seated fourth glute work, 114–115
    shoulder slides (fitness ball), 220–221
    side lifts (fitness ball), 222–223

T–U–V